Healthy Body,
Better Birthing

Healthy Body, Better Birthing

Francesca Naish and Janette Roberts

Newleaf

Published in Ireland 2001 by
Newleaf
an imprint of
Gill & Macmillan Ltd
Hume Avenue, Park West, Dublin 12
with associated companies throughout the world
www.gillmacmillan.ie

0 7171 3217 X

Printed by ColourBooks Ltd, Dublin

Copyright © Francesca Naish and Janette Roberts 2000

First published in Australia and New Zealand in 2000 under
the title, *The Natural Way to Better Birth and Bonding*,
by Doubleday, Australia an imprint of Transworld
Publishers Division of Random House Australia

A CIP catalogue record for this book is available from the British Library.

1 3 5 4 2

The information provided in this book is intended for general
information and guidance only, and this should not be used as
a substitute for consulting a qualified health practitioner.
Neither the authors nor the publishers can accept any
responsibility for your health or any side-effects of
treatments described in this book.

Contents

About the authors

About Francesca

Francesca Naish was born in England in 1946. She studied mathematics at Sussex University but, after arrival in Australia, when in her late twenties, established a Natural Birth Control practice in Paddington, Sydney. This grew into The Village Healing and Growth Centre, one of the first holistic health-care practices in Australia. Since 1994 she has trained health professionals in the use of her unique Natural Fertility Management techniques including 'Better Babies' preconception health care, and has recently established agencies in New Zealand, Malaysia, the United States and England. In 1995, after 20 years in clinical practice, she established The Jocelyn Centre in Woollahra, Sydney. This is the first clinic in Australia to specialise in natural methods for fertility management, reproductive health and preconception health care.

Francesca is a qualified naturopath, herbalist and hypnotherapist. She writes extensively for the press, appears regularly on radio and television and is sought after as a public speaker and lecturer. She also pioneered the teaching in Australia of natural vision improvement. She has written four previous books: *The Lunar Cycle* (1989), *Natural Fertility* (1991), *The Natural Way to Better Babies: Preconception Health Care for Prospective Parents* (1996) and *The Natural Way to a Better Pregnancy* in 1999. The last two books were co-authored with Janette Roberts, and 'Better Babies' is now published as *Healthy*

Parents, Better Babies in the USA and UK. Francesca has two sons and lives in the Sydney suburb of Bronte with her family.

About Janette

Janette was born in Sydney in 1947 and graduated from Sydney University with an Honours degree in Pharmacy in 1968. Her career as a community pharmacist spanned almost twenty years, but a growing interest in nutritional and environmental medicine led her to complete a Postgraduate Diploma in Clinical Nutrition in 1983. She retired from pharmacy before the birth of her first son in 1985, but by then she had developed a specific interest in preconception health care, which she has promoted in Australia on behalf of the British Foresight Association since 1987. Her first book *The Natural Way to Better Babies: Preconception Health Care for Prospective Parents* (co-authored with Francesca Naish) was published in 1996. It is now published as *Healthy Parents, Better Babies* in the USA and UK. This title was followed by *The Natural Way to a Better Pregnancy* in 1999.

Janette makes frequent appearances on radio and television, and presents public lectures to prospective parents and workshops and seminars to health professionals around Australia and New Zealand. In 1998 she and two partners established Balmain Wellness Centre which offers programs for anti-ageing, vitality, longevity and care before conception and during pregnancy. It is situated in the Sydney suburb of Balmain where Janette lives with her two sons.

Acknowledgements

Janette's acknowledgements

As a young woman I was a passionate atheist with an equally passionate commitment to remaining childless . . . aah, the arrogance and folly of one's youth. As a much wiser woman, entering the second half-century of my life, I constantly feel the presence of a great power at work behind the scenes and have an acute awareness of the Divine hand in every aspect of our lives. My greatest debt of gratitude must be to that power responsible for turning my commitment to childlessness into an equally heartfelt commitment to having children, and to conceiving, giving birth to and nurturing them as Nature intended. That same power has also given me the opportunity to tell my story and to encourage women to do as I did. I am humbled by the opportunity and in awe of the great wisdom of that guiding hand.

On a more practical level, my mother always believed in what I was doing, even though what I did with my children was vastly different from what she did with hers. Stan, all women should have a mother as supportive! The father of my children, despite initial scepticism, supported my birthing and breastfeeding choices. Alexander, it was good to share the family bed. My midwife helped me truly experience the wonder of pregnancy, birth, bonding and breastfeeding, and many years ago made a written contribution to this book. Sue, swe finally made it into print. CAPERS (a Queensland organisation which disseminates information about all aspects of child-bearing) encouraged my public speaking and my writing, and sold my books. Jan, thanks for all your support along the way. The executive director of Lamaze International allowed me to reproduce its tips for choosing a childbirth educator. Linda, many thanks. Once again, the director of Castlemaine Iyengar Studio has advised us on appropriate yoga poses. Cheryl, it's time to write your own book. Many women have written on the subject of birth, and many more have related their birth experiences (good and bad). To you all, thanks for sharing your stories.

Akal Khalsa came with help on the first morning of my second son's life, when things weren't going quite the way we'd planned. Michael's story is found within these pages and Akal supported me generously then, just as she supports me now. In the throes of resuming her career as a homebirth midwife, she has taken the time to offer her thoughts on the manuscript. Akal, I am enormously grateful for your input and wish you and all your birthing families much joy and happiness.

Our agent, recently a new mother herself, has managed to attend to our affairs as well as her infant son. Liz, thanks for all your endeavours on our behalf, and for sharing your thoughts on Caesarean birth. Our editors at Random House have been unflinching in their support and understanding. Fiona, Katie and Amanda, our book is a tribute to your enthusiasm and patience. Our beautiful cover girl and her baby daughter are an embodiment of all we write about. Francesca and Isabella, thank you for allowing us to capture your love and your light on film. Pedantry and nit-picking have their day. Barry, thank you for your help with the proofreading (and for everything else too).

When my co-author and I embarked on writing *The Natural Way to Better Babies* we never imagined that four sequels would be commissioned, nor foresaw the success of the series in overseas markets. We certainly never imagined that a pharmacist and naturopath would be writing on subjects for which they have no more training than that received on the spot as women and mothers. Yet we are constantly amazed at the flow of ideas and words that never seems to stop. Dear Francesca, you've taught me heaps and we've had a load of laughs. But I beg you, please stop sending me all that information for inclusion in an already oversized manuscript, and please, please learn to use a computer and the Internet!

Finally, my powerful past-life connection and partner, this time around, in Balmain Wellness Centre is, as he has always been, enthusiastic, encouraging and supportive. He understands my absences from our joint venture as I attend to deadlines. He infuses me with a total belief in myself and goads me to achieve more than I ever thought possible. He shares my passion for all those subjects that have captured my imagination and tirelessly indulges my endless ideas and flights of fancy. He brings me inspiration, equilibrium and transformation. Billy, thank you for more than you will ever know.

Francesca's acknowledgements

Like Janette, I came to childbearing relatively late in life and had previously sworn that children were not for me. But then, whatever goddess, primal force or biological imperative it is that creates the urge to reproduce grabbed me with both hands and I knew nothing else would happen in my life until I had done this thing. And so my most heartfelt thankfulness, like Janette's, is to this force which transformed me into a mother—the most profoundly joyful and humbling experience of my life. Much of my working life is spent helping other women and couples to achieve this experience and their profound joy is a continuing inspiration, so my thanks go to them as well.

My own birthing experiences (as you will read later) were complicated by a pelvic injury sustained in my youth. But the midwives and doctors assisting me gave their unstinting support, and my thanks go to them for their part in those two intense experiences, which still burn brightly in my memory despite the problems we overcame. They enabled me to be more flexible in my approach to the way we birth our children.

My associates and colleagues at the Jocelyn Centre for Natural Fertility Management are always due immense gratitude for their sharing of knowledge and their support, which makes it possible for me to take the time to write. Also deserving a mention are all those involved in Natural Fertility Management who help spread the good word that it is possible to approach all those parts of our lives which are to do with fertility naturally and with confidence.

I join Jan in her acknowledgements of our wonderful agent, editors and cover girl, and I'd also like to join her in thanking Akal Khalsa for her invaluable input. Many thanks also to Anna Brennan for sharing her thoughts on post-natal depression; to Vicki Turner-Wolfe for her help with the homoeopathic remedies; to Miriam Camara for her advice on the acupuncture points; to my NFM student for the story of her experiences with the lunar cycle, conceptions and births; to Nicole Mason for typing the manuscript; and to Sarah Parsons for her invaluable support in keeping the Jocelyn Centre running as I hide away to write.

To Malcolm, the father of my children, who has shared with me the joy of parenting, and to my dear sons, Albion and Sebastian, who enrich my life immeasurably, go my love and gratitude. Without them I would never have trodden this path.

Finally, thanks to my dear co-author, Janette, who helps me keep my sense of humour when deadlines loom and who is a constant source of inspiration to keep writing. When I read what she has written, I know our public will enjoy it as much as I do.

Note to readers

In this book we deal with both self-help and practitioner-guided treatments. If you are in any doubt about what you should do on your own or what requires professional help, always seek help. But be sure that the medical advice you receive is from a practitioner who has a commitment to using as natural and non-interventionist an approach as possible.

The herbs and supplements that we recommend will be available from a number of different sources including holistic and natural health practitioners, health food stores and pharmacies. Supermarkets also carry an increasing range of supplements and remedies, but wherever you purchase your products, make sure that they fulfil the dosages that we recommend.

In the case of nutritional supplements we have given clear guidelines regarding dosages for general use. Herbal and other natural remedies come in a variety of forms, and it is therefore not possible to give similarly clear-cut guidelines for dosage. Whether the product is a tablet, capsule, loose herb, fluid extract or powder, if it is sold through a retail outlet it will have clear directions for use on the container and you should follow those. If you are in any doubt or if you have specific concerns it is always advisable to consult a natural health practitioner. You can take a copy of our book to your practitioner for reference.

Throughout the text we have referred to your baby as 'he'. We would like to reassure you that our only reason for doing so is to distinguish easily between references to the mother and the baby. Though neither of us has been fortunate enough to have a daughter we would certainly have welcomed such an addition to our brood of delightful sons.

Foreword

Thoughts from Janette

In 1984 I was managing a retail pharmacy in Sydney's CBD. Over the previous few years I had become increasingly involved in the practice of nutritional and environmental medicine, interested in preconception health care in particular, and less and less committed to continuing my career (which then spanned seventeen years) in pharmacy. I had also decided, after many years of saying 'no children', that as my fortieth birthday loomed ever closer, it was now or never. Then one of those synchronicities, which occur in all our lives, and which we attend to with varying degrees of attention (or inattention), occurred in mine.

During the previous months I had observed the burgeoning pregnant belly of a beautiful woman of Indian descent who was a customer in the pharmacy. My interest wasn't especially avid, because I'd never been particularly interested in the state of pregnancy, but I was aware of a wonderful energy about this woman and her partner. When she finally appeared one day with their absolutely exquisite newborn nestled at her breast, I casually asked her if she had had a good birth.

With hindsight I am still amazed that I asked the question. What constituted a 'good' birth (or its opposite) was not something I was familiar with. As far as I knew then, the sort of birth one experienced wasn't high on the list of things that really mattered. Compared to what I now know of such things, what I knew at that moment in my life amounted to zip! However, I am now absolutely certain that when I asked that question it was the great omnipotent hand which guides all our lives giving some very firm direction to mine.

You may have already guessed the woman's answer. She told me that her baby daughter had been born at home. Her simple statement hit me like a lightning bolt. Instantly, I knew that was what I wanted to do—give birth to my children at home. Consider that I had not yet even tried to conceive, had only recently (at the grand old age of 37) come to the realisation that I really wanted to become a mother, and was not, until that instant, even aware that births could take place at home. Yet my absolute certainty of the rightness of such an undertaking was completely overwhelming.

That certainty has led me on a journey of discovery which has changed the shape and direction of my whole life. It has led me to question not only where, but how, when and with whom women give birth to their babies. It has also caused me to examine every aspect of reproduction and child raising and the many ways in which they are now under constant surveillance, medically managed or just plain interfered with.

I already knew something of the adverse affects of our twentieth-century diet, lifestyle and environment on our general health. When I began to read more widely I discovered that these factors also adversely affected fertility, pregnancy and the birth, bonding and breastfeeding processes. These perfectly normal, natural functions were further compromised by medical management. Along with the increase in surveillance, management and intervention there had been a parallel decline in the degree to which women relied on their intuition when raising their children. Maternal instincts were often absent, and when present, frequently ignored.

What began as a glimpse of enlightenment became a much clearer view after I had conceived, given birth to and nurtured two children of my own. All of these things, including the miscarriage of a third child, were done in ways that were well outside the present social and cultural norm, but they were done in ways that reflected much earlier traditions. I raised my children in much the same way that, once, all women did such things. I practised 'immersion mothering,' or 'natural nurturing,' and in doing so realised that some very fundamental things had been forgotten and many more lost in our amorous embrace of scientific progress, technological wizardry and trendy psychological theory. My sons are now 14 and 9 years old, and as they have grown and developed that view has become clearer still, and with it, my desire to share those views, and in doing so, perhaps to offer a small measure of enlightenment to others.

Thoughts from Francesca

Like Jan, my birthing stories have their share of the divine. However, the goddess who was directing the birth of my first child definitely had a sense of humour—and some of the jokes were on me. The lessons I learnt from this, and the different choices I then made, gave me insights into how important it is to know what you want, to know how to get it, to know what questions to ask, and to know what your options are. I hope this book will go some way to making those choices easier for you.

Like Jan, I left conception until a time in my life which, in those days, was relatively late. I had no thoughts of pregnancy or children until I was 27, then became gradually more obsessed with it until I decided that this desire would not go away and had to be fulfilled. I was lucky enough to conceive easily on the day I had chosen as most auspicious—that this happened to be Friday 13th should have given me pause, but since my life had always been ruled by the bizarre, this seemed no exception. (My son, who arrived six weeks early on April Fools' Day, seems to have had a sense of humour thrust upon him from the outset.)

I had no thoughts of problems, I was dedicated to a healthy life-style, had practised natural birth control before conception, and was practising natural medicine. My pregnancy went like a dream, as I knew it would, and I almost forgot that there were potential problems from a serious pelvic injury that I had sustained in a car accident when I was 20. However, this awareness was sufficient for me to be wary of choosing a home birth, living as I was in the mountains, quite far from the nearest town.

Unfortunately, birthing centres were not then available, so I sought out the best option on offer, a highly regarded doctor who practised 'Le Boyer' techniques—a soft entry for the baby into the world cushioned by water, dim lighting and subdued noise. It never occurred to me that the birth would be anything other than perfect, as my pregnancy had been.

When my son started to arrive six weeks prematurely as a result of my pelvic problems, all hopes of a gentle birth were lost. I became aware how ill-prepared I was to understand, cope with or have input into the decisions and actions that followed. All control was wrested from me, and all manner of drugs pumped into me. My son was born drunk (from an alcohol drip to which I was attached), and I was confused and exhausted.

The intense joy of mothering soon wiped out those feelings, but I was aware that I would never really know whether what he and I had experienced was truly inevitable, or whether, if I had been better prepared, things could have been managed better.

For the birth of my second son, I did things differently. This was made easier for me by the existence of a wonderful birthing centre at the local maternity hospital, staffed by midwives whom I got to know well. By then I was deeply involved in my Natural Fertility Management practice, and had a better understanding of the available resources. My obstetrician was a gentle, caring man who had a home-birth practice, an affinity with natural medicine and respected the skills of the midwives.

This time I managed to 'hold on' to my baby until full term. However, my damaged pelvis still affected my ability to give birth, and, after a promising start, the labour did not progress well and my carers decided that the baby was stuck and in distress. Although I ended up with an epidural and forceps delivery (and a baby who had the cord wrapped twice around his neck), I was part of the decision-making process all along, and confident that my carers knew of my preferences and were advising me with this in mind. As a consequence, I felt fully involved and in control. Though the outcome was not my preferred option, I had made informed choices. For me, this transformed the process and the way I felt about it.

This is what we want you to receive from this book. There is no right way to give birth, and there may be many surprises in store. But if you have information, if you have sought out carers who understand and support you and your choices, if you have prepared well and given yourself the best possible chance of achieving your goals, then there will be no regrets.

As I had taken care before conception and during pregnancy to eat well, avoid all toxins and generally live a healthy lifestyle, my sons were both born with robust health. Consequently, they were little affected by these experiences, though my first son suffers a very mild degree of dyslexia which is common to those who have experienced difficult births. My chosen mode of mothering, with full and extended breastfeeding and continual mother–child contact, continued to support my boys and their progress as 'better babies'.

My experiences have left me with the abiding belief that you can't leave something as important as the birth of your child to chance. Whatever your eventual experience it can be positive if you are confident that you are making the best possible choices open to you, and that your carers and guides are sympathetic to your preferences.

Public awareness of natural birthing is greater than it ever was, but so is the pressure to conform to a medical model. All your 'better babies' will arrive in their own way, but your support of them from before conception through to weaning and your choice of natural, safe alternatives whenever possible are what we hope to encourage through this and all our 'Better Babies' books.

Thoughts from both of us

In 1994 we were not even personally acquainted, although we were each aware of the work that the other was doing. Then Francesca was approached by Random House to write a book on preconception health care. She agreed, if she could do it in conjunction with Jan. Our first face-to-face meeting was certainly one of those divinely inspired events. Our earlier books *The Natural Way to Better Babies* and *The Natural Way to a Better Pregnancy* discuss the factors adversely affecting fertility, pregnancy and foetal and infant health. Those adverse effects are largely the result of the changes that humankind has wrought in the environment and of the unhealthy lifestyle habits that have been adopted over the last two hundred years. But it's not enough to describe those adverse effects, nor enough to tell you that most pregnancies and babies could be 'better'. Our books detail very simply all the steps you need to take to ensure that you have a 'better pregnancy' and a truly 'better baby', as well as explaining how very important it is that you do so.

This book is simply an extension of those two earlier books. The same dietary, lifestyle and environmental factors which compromise the health of both pregnancies and babies have also caused a deterioration in the ease with which women give birth. Furthermore, medical intervention in a perfectly normal, healthy, physical function has made labour and birth more of an ordeal than a major and memorable life event for a significant number of women. A further consequence of these same factors is the interruption of the mother–infant bond, which has implications extending far beyond the mother–baby relationship. But again, knowing that our meddling with nature has compromised both birth and bonding isn't enough, so this book gives you lots of ideas for putting things to rights.

We hope that what we have to say will put the act of giving birth back into its proper perspective as a perfectly normal function. When a birth is allowed to proceed normally, supported by empathetic birth attendants, it becomes an empowering and transformative life event, rather than an endurance test. When the bonding between mother and baby also unfolds naturally, the positive effects extend way beyond the immediate family. 'Better birth' and 'better bonding' are simply birth and bonding as nature intended them to be, and despite the pervasiveness of the medical model having both is not an impossibility, but can be quite easily achieved with some forethought and prior knowledge of exactly what each involves.

To all the midwives through the centuries

The experience of birth

The most appropriate environment in which to give birth is that in which you make love. In earlier generations, women usually gave birth in the place in which their child was conceived. This was a familiar place; not always a spacious or elegant place, often not even a particularly clean place, but a place where they felt completely comfortable and very much at ease.

For millennia, women gave birth at home with the support and encouragement of other women. Midwives, doulas and close women acquaintances would offer physical comfort, emotional support and talk a woman through her labour. Their wisdom, based on practical experience and handed down through generations, took full account of a mother's intuitive feelings. They would also remain with her after the birth to nurture her in the early postpartum days, to keep her and her newborn baby safe, secluded and well-nourished in the weeks before the new mother resumed her regular activities.

Traditionally, when women gave birth they did so with a profound understanding and acceptance of the normality of the process. From the time they were young girls they had seen and heard births taking place around them. As teenagers and young women they had almost certainly been present when relatives or close friends gave birth. They didn't see it as something abnormal, let alone pathological, and certainly didn't consider it cause for interference.

MODERN BIRTHS: WHAT IS MISSING?

The majority of women in Western society today give birth in places and situations far removed from those conducive to intimacy. Not only is it impossible for a strange environment, such as a hospital, to be intimate, but many women now labour virtually alone, hooked up only to the cold comfort of electronic machinery. The vigilant watching and waiting, and the constant presence of a caring and compassionate human being, is replaced by the impersonality of monitoring machines. While midwives are still present at births, their role has changed. Some are little more than an obstetrician's handmaiden and others frequently too busy to be able to give the one-to-one comfort and the continuity of encouragement, counselling and support which is essential for new mothers. Women frequently give birth amongst, and spend their early postpartum days surrounded by, people who are strangers.

These days, the woman who has seen another woman give birth before she gives birth herself is a rare exception. 'Preparation for childbirth' classes are an attempt to replace the hands-on, experiential learning which, once, most women got automatically. While many of these classes are run by supportive, caring and empathetic individuals, with a real understanding of the feelings and needs of birthing women and their babies, many others are little more than a preparation for a high-tech delivery in a hospital setting. As well, most women giving birth today would consider themselves fortunate if they have ever seen a baby breastfeeding. In fact, many may never have held a newborn in their arms.

That wonderful pool of women's knowledge which encompassed all sorts of birthing, feeding and nurturing practices and was handed down through generations is no longer available. It has been replaced by advice from a variety of 'experts' who have no such ancient wisdom to impart to women. Their offerings are often platitudes and inaccuracies, dispensed in the name of scientific progress. Yet women are frequently in awe of these so-called experts. Seduced by degrees and titles, they may follow advice that goes against their better judgement, and ignores their maternal instinct. Occasionally women may be so confused that they cannot even identify their intuitive, instinctive feelings, much less heed them.

Yet intimacy, support, and an abundance of well-tried advice and information are essential for new mothers. They are the ingredients for a fulfilling birth which gives women a sense of wholeness and personal worth as well as feelings of real achievement. They contribute to a bonding experience that gives them a sense of oneness and connection with their babies that affects every aspect of their future parenting.

Perhaps you're thinking *'Well, what the hell? Intimacy, support and old midwives just had to go. Births are now very safe. Women no longer lose their lives, they no longer have to suffer the pain, and babies who would once have died, now survive. Surely this is what progress is all about?'*

If the foregoing statement reflects your thinking, then our book is about to challenge those beliefs. Hospitals, which are an extremely recent innovation for women giving birth, have never been demonstrated to be the safest place in which to do so. Giving birth away from the hospital/medical environment is certainly not the dangerous undertaking that many consider it to be unless there is some real and unavoidable complication. In fact, the countries in the developed world that have the lowest rate of neo-natal mortality are those countries that have the highest rate of births occurring at home.

Today, in our society, fewer women die in childbirth than in the past, but many suffer unnecessary physical, mental and emotional trauma of varying degrees. The pain of childbirth can now be completely alleviated, but that pain is not necessarily a bad thing and may actually have some beneficial effects. As well, many serious questions are now being asked about our present ability to save all but the most extremely premature infants. While there are certainly advantages in a medically managed birth for very high-risk pregnancies and deliveries, we believe that the radical changes in birthing practices, which now extend to almost all women, have been regressive rather than the reverse.

These changes in birth practices, from an intimate, woman-centred event to a largely male-dominated, medical procedure have occurred in the space of a blink of the eye in evolutionary terms. It is not possible, therefore, to identify clearly all of the ill effects for which these changes are responsible. But we believe that tampering with the birth and bonding processes has profound implications for the physical, mental and emotional health of families, and ultimately for the society in which we live. By making you aware of how far-reaching are the consequences of this meddling, we hope to encourage you to take responsibility for having a 'better birth' and 'better bonding.'

What both these terms encompass are those traditional practices that served women and their babies well for thousands of generations. They simply involve a return to old ways and eschew the embrace of intervention in these completely normal processes, leaving medical technology to its valid role as emergency medicine. Let's take a look now at the 'old ways', and what was good about them—then discover how and why they were changed. Then we'll show you how these changes may not be for the better.

THE HISTORY OF CHILDBIRTH

Statistics tell us that 90 per cent of women are able to have a perfectly normal, uncomplicated labour and delivery without any assistance or outside interference. Yet those who actually manage to do so, represent only a very small fraction of this number. Today, many women think that high-tech monitoring and obstetrical interventions offer them significant advantages. They also believe that giving birth is a much safer undertaking if it occurs in a hospital. These beliefs are still relatively widespread, although we're happy to say that they're changing. The history of the medicalisation of labour and childbirth provides some insights into how this belief pattern arose and also looks at the changes which are currently taking place.

Traditional midwifery

The practice of midwifery goes back as far as recorded history. The word midwife means 'with woman' and as long as women have been giving birth, there have been midwives. Traditionally, through thousands of generations, births were the exclusive province of women and giving birth was seen as a normal, healthy event. No one doubted that a woman, left to labour at her own pace, was perfectly capable of bringing her baby into the world with very little outside help. Women's bodies were considered well designed to bear children—a fact attested to by the burgeoning human population that has been largely achieved without medical intervention.

In traditional or tribal societies the midwife had various aids to assist a woman in labour. These might have included herbal infusions or special foods. Essential oils may have been heated and inhaled, or used as part of a massage routine. Whether it was herbs, or other treatments that were administered, all had a long tradition of safe use. Women in these cultures always laboured in an upright position. Squatting was the position usually favoured for the delivery of the baby. A log, a block of wood, a stout pole, or a rope helped a woman maintain the squat, and other women may also have lent physical support. Birthing stools were also common, and illustrations of these devices and others used in labour, as well as depictions of labouring and birthing positions are found in many cultures dating back thousands of years. There is an ancient Egyptian hieroglyph meaning 'birth' which depicts a woman squatting on stones, and numerous clay statues, temple carvings, marble figurines and pieces of jewellery from Copper-Age Turkish, Aztec, Chinese, Japanese and early Greek and Roman cultures depict active births.

In these older, traditional societies, the midwife was well respected and her advice sought for all sorts of things, apart from those associated with pregnancy, birth and breastfeeding. She was usually well-versed in traditional herbal lore. She was also wise in the ways of the earth and its natural rhythms, in tune with seasonal changes and cycles of birth, death and rebirth. She certainly understood something of the movements of the sun, the moon and the planets and of their effects on crops as well as people. In those few tribal societies that still flourish, her role as midwife, medicine woman and healer is probably largely unchanged today.

However, in some cultures, even though the practice of midwifery was extremely well established (and was well outside the practice of medicine), midwives aroused strong passions. From the late fifteenth until well into the seventeenth century, many European and English midwives practised at risk of their lives. Seen as inquiring, independent spirits, with access to material such as umbilical cords, amniotic sacs and placentas (which were all considered to have magical properties), midwives represented a threat to church and state. Many were burnt at the stake for their practices and 'black arts'. Even when the witch-hunts abated, midwives were left tainted, and were generally referred to in derogatory terms.

Take Sairy Gamp for example. The drunken, inept midwife depicted in Charles Dickens' *Martin Chuzzlewit*—'*whose nose in particular was somewhat red and swollen . . . She went to a lying-in or a laying-out with equal zest and relish'*—could have been a prototype for the many incompetent, drunken, health practitioners of the day. However, midwives alone were singled out for adverse comment, and spoken of as if the infamous Gamp was the norm. One English medical historian, Anthony Smith, writes of midwives as '*ragged old harridans who travelled from house to house like tinkers with their old-fashioned labour chair and filthy hooks hanging from their belts*' and conveniently ignores the long history of English midwifery. Not surprisingly, given this previous bad press, many individuals are still suspicious of midwives, herbalists and other natural health practitioners today.

The rise of male birth attendants

Encroachment into the territory of birth, which had always been that of women, began in England in the thirteenth century with the rise of the barber–surgeon guilds. The right to use surgical instruments belonged exclusively to the surgeon, and if a birth failed to progress the midwife called him in and he performed an embryotomy. This involved crushing the foetal skull, dismembering the baby, and removing it piece by piece from the mother's body. Alternatively, if the mother died, the surgeon was called to perform a Caesarean section to save the baby. Obviously, this very early medical–surgical involvement in the birth process never resulted in a live baby from a live mother.

Male involvement in the birth process gained ground as men turned what started off as a trade into a lucrative profession. Remember, this only occurred because the tools of trade were their exclusive province, and without them it is doubtful whether we would ever have seen the rise of interventionist obstetrics.

In the 1500s, the surgeons to the Kings of France began to teach the methods of extraction and version (turning the baby while in the womb). When this was successful it allowed for the birth of a child who was lying sideways in the uterus. However, it was firmly believed that women did not have the physical strength, or intellect, to perform this manoeuvre and it remained for men *'with minds more alert than women's'* to carry it out.

In the late sixteenth century, Peter Chamberlen developed the first obstetrical forceps. His invention was kept a family secret for over a century as the Chamberlens used all sorts of subterfuges, including blindfolding family members present at a birth, to keep their specialist device from prying eyes.

About 1720, when the secret of the construction of these forceps at last became known, there was an explosion in their use by male midwives. Interestingly, not all practitioners were in favour of indiscriminate use, with one physician known to remark, *'The better the midwife, the thicker the rust.'* Not surprisingly, more women died at the hands of these male accoucheurs with their instruments than ever died at the hands of female midwives, who delivered babies using only their hands.

Despite this, the number of births attended by men continued to grow, due in no small part to the fact that male birth attendants charged higher fees and were therefore equated with higher social status. ('So what's new?' you might ask.) As well, there was an increasing need for intervention during the eighteenth and nineteenth centuries when there was a rise in the number of problem deliveries. This decline in the ease with which women gave birth was due to the frequency with which they had children coupled with their very poor diets.

This period corresponded with the introduction of the refining of grains. Refining brought with it deficiencies of essential minerals such as zinc, magnesium and manganese and the B-complex vitamins. Rickets (due to lack of calcium and vitamin D) was also common and this led to deformity of the pelvis and a further decrease in the efficiency of the birth process. There is some feeling too, that the very tightly laced corsets which many women favoured at this time may have contributed to the rise in the number of long, difficult labours.

While there was certainly an increased demand for the services of the male birth-attendants, there is no doubt that many surgical interventions were unnecessary and many of them also caused a great deal of damage. However the attendants became adept at concealing injuries and errors *'with a cloud of hard words and scientific jargon'*. With at least twenty modern obstetrical interventions known to be harmful, and iatrogenic (doctor-induced) complications costing the lives of 2400 babies in the UK every year, you might be forgiven for asking 'What's changed?' But this *'meddlesome midwifery,'* as it became known, was the forerunner of the many and varied obstetrical interventions we see today.

During the 1700s, an increased knowledge of anatomy and physiology saw surgeons involved in formal midwifery training, from which women were excluded. These doctors saw the opportunity to expand their practices by attending women in labour. Once they had done so, the woman and her family would frequently be their patients forever. However, the training and skill of these doctors was of an extremely variable standard, and, despite this training, the first example in the UK of a Caesarean section in which both mother and baby survived was attributed to an illiterate Irish midwife.

The grasp which the male medical attendants had on the birth process was further strengthened when they gained access to anaesthesia during the mid-nineteenth century. Queen Victoria was the first woman in England to use chloroform while giving birth and it is certain that this embrace of a new medical development by royalty heightened its desirability.

The male attendants' ability to ease pain with chloroform and to shorten the duration of labour with forceps meant a further increase in the number of men attending births. Of course, both forceps deliveries and the use of chloroform ensured that women were on their backs and confined to bed while giving birth and it wasn't long before this practice spread throughout the Western world.

The move to hospital births

The 1920s–50s saw a change in the domestic environment culminating in gleaming porcelain kitchens and bathrooms with an unnatural emphasis on cleanliness. The sterile hospital setting with masks, gowns, strict attention to hygiene, feeding schedules, and other inflexible routines paralleled this change in living standards. In the early days of hospital deliveries pregnant women were treated as if they were 'sick' and were given general anaesthesia. The delivery room was the operating theatre and the obstetrician was a surgeon. The recumbent position was further refined to the lithotomy position (feet up in stirrups). While this was physiologically unsound for the woman giving birth it made things convenient for the doctor. It meant he didn't have to get down on his hands and knees to check the progress of labour.

Even though the male attendants, and then doctors, had initially carved out their niche at those births that were problematic, eventually all births came to be viewed as pathological and the incorporation of the birth process into the medical model was complete. At the same time, practices of infant feeding and nurturing were changing and the use of artificial formulae and scheduled feeds was on the rise.

So by the early twentieth century, medicine had gained complete control over the birthing population. The autonomy of midwives was in decline. In 1902, when the Central Midwifery Board was established in the USA, it had no mandatory midwives' representative. (It wasn't until 1973 that a midwife became chairperson!) Midwives simply became assistants to obstetricians and gynaecologists, even though it was never established that midwifery care was inferior.

THE MODERN MEDICAL MODEL

The medical model of birth is about control, power and authority. It is a view of birth that is symptomatic of the patriarchal society. Obstetricians and gynaecologists, who are mostly male, have a man's eye view of women's bodies. The male body is perceived as normal and consequently pregnancy and birth are (at best) stresses on the system. At worst, they are disease states. Women have been considered 'unwell', 'indisposed', 'in a delicate condition' and so on.

Doctors, in most instances, also subscribe to the mind–body split. Obstetric texts refer to the 'maternal pelvis', the 'contracting uterus' and the 'dilating cervix' without once referring to the mind which is attached to these body parts. A similar dualism means that the baby and mother are viewed as a dichotomy when they are, in fact, an integral unit.

Furthermore, the medical model reflects the technological mind-set of society that views the body as a machine. A birthing body can be made to perform more efficiently—it can be made faster and quieter.

These interventions in the birthing process might be likened to someone endlessly fine tuning a television set, while all the time it is connected to the wrong antenna.

What's more, obstetricians and gynaecologists are trained to manage complications. They are specialists in the abnormal, their training focuses almost entirely on what can go wrong. Very few observe the huge range of variations that constitutes normal birth. They feel completely powerless, perhaps even threatened, in a situation which is best managed by watching and waiting. They feel compelled to act.

They see the pain of childbirth solely in terms of their ability to relieve it. In reality, the pain (at the risk of glorifying what really and truly does hurt) might more profitably be viewed as a rite of passage to motherhood and (as we will explore in Chapter 7) a series of cues to the labouring woman, letting her understand and manage the progress of her baby's birth.

However we must be fair and point out that doctors have not been entirely responsible for wanting to ease the pain of childbirth, or for wanting to speed things up and help things along. The general population and many individuals (including birthing women) have become increasingly inclined to abrogate responsibility for their own health and wellbeing. They are enamoured of a comfortable pain-free existence and a quick fix. They also subscribe to the mind-set that considers the doctor or the hospital responsible for the quality of their birth experience and the health and wellbeing of their baby. We even know of women (otherwise reasonably active in their own health management) who opt for an elective Caesarean, just to avoid the possible pain or hassle of a natural birth.

Of course, obstetricians vary a great deal. These days there are many more who are sympathetic to a natural and non-interventionist approach to birth. Those registered with birthing centres are likely to be amongst them.

A RETURN TO TRADITION?

While most doctors and their patients were avidly embracing the seductive, modern, medical model, there was a swing away from total management of the birth process. In 1933 in the UK, Grantly Dick Read made some observations of birthing women and concluded that '*If fear can be eliminated, pain will cease'*. This stemmed from the now famous remark, made to him by a woman in labour, *'It didn't hurt! It wasn't meant to, was it doctor?'* Grantly Dick Read emphasised the need for constant emotional support for the labouring woman and though his work was well received in the UK, it was less popular in the USA where it didn't fit very well in the hospital environment. (While we agree that eliminating the baseless fears that have sprung up around childbirth with the ascendancy of the medical model is essential if women are to experience a better birth, we would not go so far as to claim that pain will also completely disappear! But pain can certainly be managed without recourse to drugs—see Chapter 7.)

In 1951, in the Soviet Union, work was being done on Pavlovian responses. Lamaze, a French doctor, studied these methods and in 1956 he published his book *Painless Childbirth*. He advocated that the uterine contractions were stimuli to which different responses could be learned. Fear and pain could be unlearned. His techniques, which tried to give women back some sense of control when they gave birth, were much better accepted into the hospital setting than those of Read. However, both Read and Lamaze were instrumental in alerting women to the fact that there was more to birth than being drugged out of their minds and waking up only when their baby was washed, weighed and wearing a clean nappy.

Frederick LeBoyer, a French obstetrician, also had a major impact on birthing practices. He delivered nine thousand babies by conventional methods, but then began to ponder the reasons for the high proportion of dysfunctional children in France. He journeyed to India where he studied traditional birthing methods then returned to his native country and put his ideas into practice. A LeBoyer birth occurs in a quiet room, away from bright lights, the cord is not cut immediately and afterwards the baby is immersed in a warm bath and is then gently massaged.

Babies born in this way appeared to be more alert, smiling and content compared to their more roughly handled contemporaries, some of whom were still being held upside down and slapped on their bottoms. Although not all births were, or are, able to follow this exact pattern, LeBoyer's ideas have had a substantial influence on our understanding of the possible effects of a traumatic birth and on the ways they can be reduced.

Another step forward—and one that broke with tradition—occurred in the 1970s. Fathers were allowed to be present at the birth of their child. (Dick Read had advocated this change as early as the 1940s and 1950s, although few hospitals had acted on his advice.) However, even when they were finally admitted, they were usually no more than an observer in a sterile gown, in awe of the whole process, and often asked to leave the room if things got a bit 'sticky'. But it meant there was a chink in the hospital armour—and that chink has been growing steadily wider ever since. These days the father that chooses not to be present when his partner gives birth is considered a rare exception rather than the reverse.

Now, at the beginning of the twentieth-first century there is increasing recognition that women have been short-changed in allowing themselves to be 'managed' through the transformative life event of giving birth. Enlightened birth practitioners and consumers everywhere are seeking to change the status quo. They want birth to be a normal and wonderfully joyful part of a woman's life, not a pathological event to be feared and endured only with medical assistance. There is also a small but growing tendency away from males attending births. Some women are recognising that giving birth is very much women's business and its power and dynamics can only be truly understood and supported fully by other women. Whether there will ever be a complete swing back to the totally women-centred event of days past remains to be seen. Given that, these days, a woman's life partner gives the support which was once offered by extended female family and friends, and fills the gaps which they have left, this may remain the choice of a minority.

Modern midwifery

With the increasing desire for women attendants at births, the situation in which midwives now find themselves throughout the world varies. In the USA, with the exception of a few progressive states, midwifery is not recognised as an independent profession. Other countries have treated their midwives more kindly and in Holland and Scandinavia they are well paid and much respected. One third of all births in Holland take place at home, and midwives are the sole attendants at more than half of that country's births. Not coincidentally, Holland has the lowest rate of neonatal and perinatal deaths in the world, and a Caesarean section rate of just 6 per cent.

The UK has always had a strong tradition of midwives attending births at home, and there, Greenwich University has established a chair in Complementary Medicine and Midwifery. The present principal lecturer at the university has an active clinical practice where she offers reflexology, aromatherapy, massage, homoeopathy and Bach flower remedies to pregnant and child-bearing women. In 1999 there was a further shift to community-based antenatal care. A year-long House of Commons inquiry into NHS maternity services was conducted. The committee stated that the assumption that giving birth in hospital is safest is unproved and that homebirths and other less medicalised options should be offered and encouraged in low-risk women.

However, Australia hasn't followed in the footsteps of the country which so largely shaped our early years. On the contrary, we seem to have embraced the American model fairly and squarely. In the 1870s, traditional midwives conducted two-thirds of all births in NSW, but by the 1930s these women had all but disappeared. It was not until the late 1970s that homebirth groups around the country became active. Despite the fact that the homebirth movement has become increasingly vocal, fewer than 0.5 per cent of births in Australia occur at home in the care of a midwife. This is not entirely surprising given the modern day witch-hunts that have been carried out against both the GPs and midwives who have attended homebirths. While burning at the stake is no longer practised, the victimisation, intimidation and, ultimately, de-registration which has been the lot of several of Australia's most prominent homebirth practitioners has been an effective deterrent to many midwives and mothers.

Across the Tasman, midwives have fought and won the battle to practise independently. In New Zealand a woman can now enroll in a degree course to study Midwifery and is no longer obliged to become a nurse first. Direct Entry Midwifery, autonomy, and the same pay as doctors are huge steps forward for New Zealand midwives and birthing women and their families in that country.

Birthing centres

Birthing centres, should, ideally, be the perfect transition, or half-way point, between homebirths and hospital births. Yet there are not nearly enough of these centres available to accommodate all the women who would like to use them. Many still have very restrictive criteria for admission, and are under the control of male obstetricians. Yet, despite the small number of homebirths occurring nationwide and despite the limited availability of birthing centres, the chances of women having completely natural, unmedicated births in intimate surroundings is not an entirely lost cause. Women's complaints about the impersonal and dehumanising aspects of birth in hospitals, the voice of the homebirth movement and the advent of birthing centres have generally had a very positive influence on the way in which hospitals treat birthing women.

In the hospitals

Many midwives, who are currently working within the traditional medical framework, are exercising their autonomy and are allowing birthing women all sorts of freedoms and options which would have been unthinkable just ten years ago. They see their role as one of watchful waiting and frequently choose not to call the doctor until the baby is born. Obstetricians are also realising that women's desire to reclaim their birth and truly experience this momentous life event is not a passing fad or an idle fancy. They realise that this movement is not something that will go away if it is ignored.

While it certainly seems unlikely that Australia will ever have a homebirth rate which approaches that of some European countries, changes are being driven by consumers, midwives and doctors working within the 'system'. Hopefully, one day, this will enable the majority of women to experience all the mystery and magic of giving birth without unnecessary management or intervention.

Which birth for you?

Just as our earlier books, *The Natural Way to Better Babies* and *The Natural Way to a Better Pregnancy* featured two stories that clearly show the difference between what we advocate and the alternative, we would like to tell you in this chapter about the difference between *a mother giving birth* and *a woman delivered of a baby*. But first, let's take a look at what (generally) happens to your body and your baby during labour and birth. What you actually experience is then largely up to you.

BEFORE LABOUR BEGINS

If you're pregnant for the first time, your baby's head will become engaged in your pelvis up to four weeks before the birth. You'll experience this as pressure in your groin and on your bladder, although you might feel that breathing is a bit easier than in the previous weeks, and there's more room under your ribs. Second and subsequent babies might not engage until labour actually begins.

As labour approaches you may also experience more frequent and intense Braxton-Hicks (or practice) contractions which rehearse your uterus for the real thing and draw up and thin (efface) the cervix. There is also an increase in the production of prostaglandins that act on the cervix, allowing it to be pulled open by the contractions, so your cervix softens and 'ripens'.

THE FIRST STAGE OF LABOUR

The first stage of labour often begins with the loss of the mucus plug from the neck of the cervix. This is called a 'show' and it will be blood stained or pinkish in colour, although this may also occur several days before true labour starts. The amniotic sac may break and the waters gush out, or there may be a slow leak of amniotic fluid. The amount of fluid lost will depend on how well engaged your baby's head is. This fluid will be constantly replenished, so those waters can't ever run dry. Quite often the amniotic sac remains intact until labour is well advanced, and occasionally the baby will be 'born in the caul' which, in olden days, was considered a good omen.

Your contractions may begin irregularly—they can feel like the dull ache of period pain—but will become stronger and closer together. You might have some diarrhoea, and vomiting is also quite likely—birth is a great emptying out, and the contents of your gut are no exception. You may be able to go back to sleep or continue with your usual activities if your labour starts slowly and contractions are spaced well apart. Some women experience a 'false' labour, with contractions starting and then stopping, before starting again. On the other hand, you may not realise that those irregular dragging sensations are doing some of the job of thinning your cervix, and when labour really gets under way, your contractions may be intense and quite close together.

Whatever gets your labour under way, or whatever signals you receive, it's important that you contact your carer when you experience any of these early signs. If you're planning to go to a birthing centre or a hospital, there's a fine balance between going too soon and being sent back home, or leaving it until you need to be completely focused on what's happening to your body. When the time comes to give those contractions all your energy and concentration you want to be secure and comfortable in the place you've chosen for the birth, not wondering if your partner's going to get you there, or your support people get to you, in time.

Once your labour is strongly established each contraction will build up to a peak and then fade away. At the peak the pain will be intense, although it is quite unlike the pain of injury. In between contractions you will have time to rest and recover. You might alternate between feeling hot and cold and, as the contractions increase in strength and the interval between them decreases, you may find yourself retreating into a sort of meditative state.

During this stage, the muscles at the top of your uterus press down on your baby's bottom and his head presses against your cervix. As he descends further into the pelvic cavity his head will rotate so that it is accommodated by the widest part of your pelvic outlet. As the descent of his head continues, it exerts pressure on your cervix, which assists dilation.

TRANSITION

This marks the end of the first stage of labour and at this point many women simply feel that they cannot continue. If you feel like that, rest assured that you're in this phase. Transition is the point when your labour reaches its peak before shifting down a gear. The strong dilating contractions are almost finished, and the bearing down stage, which is still intense, but not nearly as painful, is about to begin. Transition can be over in a flash—or it can last for an hour or two (or more) and is usually longer in a first labour. It may be the most trying part of all, and the sensations during this stage will be very powerful. Your carer will probably examine you now to see if you are fully dilated (10 cm).

THE SECOND STAGE OF LABOUR

Your baby's head is now free of your uterus and its descent and rotation continues until the crown stretches your vagina wide open. There is considerable pressure on your baby's head now, but the softness of its bones allows for this.

The contractions of second stage are quite unlike the earlier ones. These are expulsive contractions and they may begin immediately dilation is complete, or your body may need to rest if transition has been long. Even if you are feeling very tired you will be infused with new energy in second stage, as the urge to push completely overwhelms your body. Women have likened this pushing sensation to a great tidal wave that is absolutely impossible to resist. Now you will be amazed by the strength of your body as your baby is pushed down the birth canal and through the pelvic floor.

You will experience an acute burning sensation as your perineal tissues are stretched to their absolute maximum, then finally your baby's head will crown (emerge from your vagina). Then the shoulders and the rest of your baby's body will enter the world.

Newborns who have had a completely natural birth, and are then simply placed on their mother's belly, will, within 50 minutes of the birth, make their way, without any assistance whatever, to the nipple and attach themselves. This completely instinctive response is achieved using the same pushing reflex that has propelled the baby from his mother's body, and always results in 100 per cent correct attachment to the nipple.

THE THIRD STAGE OF LABOUR

Your uterus will contract and the placenta will separate from the uterine wall. Once your baby is breathing independently, the umbilical cord will stop pulsating and will be cut. (This allows the baby to receive oxygen via the placenta until his breathing is fully established.) Sometime in the first hour after the birth you will feel further contractions and the placenta (afterbirth) will be expelled. Now begins the extraordinary process of getting to know your baby.

Those are the facts facing you, an expectant mother. What will you make of them? Let's look now at the two very different births we told you about so you have some idea of the choices you'll need to make and their consequences.

STORY 1: A MOTHER GIVES BIRTH

The months of waiting, preparation and expectation are at an end. Finally this pregnant woman experiences some early contractions and a show of bloodstained mucus. She is excited when she realises that her labour is properly under way and she'll now be able to tell her own mother that this definitely isn't just a false alarm. She busies herself with some last-minute cleaning and tidying. She recognises that these chores, and others that have occupied her over the last weeks, are simply the famous nesting instinct. As the contractions strengthen and the interval between them grows shorter, she alerts her partner, her midwife and her other birth attendants.

This woman has carefully chosen a few family members and close friends to be present during her labour because she feels comfortable and secure in their presence. She feels absolutely positive about their ability to offer her their love and complete support. She has trust in them all and feels certain that no harm will come to her. Instinctively she prepares the room for the birth, putting some essential oils in a burner and scattering cushions on the floor. Weeks ago she prepared the sheets and towels she would need and they lie waiting in their brown paper wrappings.

As the contractions begin to take all this woman's concentration, she retreats to her familiar space and takes up a position on all fours, which is how, for the moment, she is most comfortable. During her pregnancy she has practised a number of positions and stretches and now she finds it easy to move from one to another as her labour progresses. She seems to know instinctively which position will help to ease the pain, which will help guide the baby into an anterior lie and which will facilitate his journey down the birth canal.

The woman stands, rocking and swaying. She sinks to her knees, rotating her pelvis. She drops to all fours, leaning forward against the bed. Her attendants massage her lower back and place hot towels on her back and belly, and later on her perineum. They offer her water to drink and help her out of her shirt when she gets hot. As the intensity of her contractions increases she moves to the shower or bath where she finds the warm water very soothing. She is free to use the toilet at any time and empties her bladder frequently. Although she vomits up the meal she ate earlier, she maintains a regular fluid intake so she won't become dehydrated, and is free to eat if she feels hungry.

In between contractions she rests and prepares herself for the next great wave of sensation that she greets with a loud groan. The sound comes from deep down inside her belly and its intensity quite surprises her. But her groaning, together with the production of endorphins, which are the body's natural pain killers, help her through the tide of pain as it ebbs and flows.

Her labour progresses at its own pace, but at no time is this woman distracted by strangers, by exploratory assessments of her progress, nor is she made anxious about the time which has elapsed. She is not apprehensive or intimidated. Her attention is focused solely on the work her body is doing. She can visualise the baby moving inexorably down the birth canal, and can imagine too, a little of the sensations that engulf him.

At last, the bag of waters breaks and the contractions increase in intensity until the woman feels she can no longer continue. As she reaches this stage, the pace of her labour changes, and shortly she is overwhelmed by the intensity of her desire to push. As she does so the pressure on her rectum causes her bowels to open, but she is not inhibited or embarrassed, just amazed at the strength and power of her body and of the all-encompassing pushing sensation. Now she takes short shallow breaths and her midwife supports her perineum as they work together to minimise any tearing.

Her midwife tells her to reach down and she can feel the exquisite softness of her baby's head as it crowns. She gives one final push and in a great orgasmic rush, the head is born. The shoulders and body slither out, covered in thick creamy vernix. 'Oh little baby, little baby!' She sees the tears in her partner's eyes, and there are tears in hers too. They are euphoric.

There is an amazing energy in the room. It transmits itself to all those present and the new parents are struck with the force and intensity of the emotion that they feel. The baby cries briefly before his mother draws him across her empty belly to her breast where he roots for her nipple and begins to suckle. In the warm room there is no sound, there are no harsh lights, but the atmosphere is charged and the mother is elated. Her sense of achievement and power know no bounds. She has never experienced anything to equal the rush of fulfilment and energy that she feels now.

The umbilical cord stops pulsing and the new father cuts it ceremoniously. At last, many minutes later, the mother experiences another contraction and the placenta is expelled. Only now do the parents look to see whether their newborn is a son or a daughter. There is laughter and amazement that this act assumes so little importance. They gaze in awe, marvelling at the perfection of their baby—the miracle of their creating.

STORY 2: A WOMAN IS DELIVERED OF HER BABY

Another expectant mother reaches the end of her pregnancy. She feels the first contractions and notices a show of bloodstained mucus. She is slightly apprehensive now that labour really seems to have begun, but soon her contractions are strong and regular and she is advised that it's time for her to go to the hospital. On arrival she is examined and found to be 2–3 cm dilated.

However, once she is out of her familiar environment, the contractions, which at home were strong and effective, become weaker. Her trip to the hospital, the admission procedures, the internal examination on arrival, and her apprehension have caused her body to produce adrenaline which is inhibiting the effect of oxytocin, the hormone which causes her uterus to contract.

She walks around, aware that it is important for her to be active, but the strength of the contractions has diminished and they are further apart. She is disappointed. The doctor, alerted that his patient is now in labour, arrives and performs another examination. He finds that the woman has advanced little from the dilation that she had achieved on admission. He decides to help things along.

He ruptures her membranes and the woman is left alone. However, once the cushioning effect of the forewaters is gone, the strength of the contractions increases and this woman, who is unprepared for the sudden and significant intensification of pain, is now afraid and soon loses control of the situation. With no one to offer her strong emotional support or alternative pain relief, she requests pain killers. Pethidine is administered, but this has little or no effect other than to make it difficult for the woman to stay awake and lucid between the contractions. Unable to gather her energy for each one, overwhelmed by their intensity that remains undiminished, she requests further pain relief.

An epidural anaesthetic is ordered. An IV infusion is set up and the mother, now numb from the waist down, is free of pain, but confined to bed. The baby reacts to the effects of the epidural. His heartbeat falters. An electrode from the CTG monitor is attached to the baby's scalp. The mother's contractions have ceased to be effective and dilation is slow. A syntocinon infusion is ordered to bring on stronger contractions.

Hours later, after receiving no nourishment or much encouragement, the woman is exhausted. She eventually reaches full dilation, but due to the effects of the epidural she is unable to push effectively. A large episiotomy is necessary. Forceps are used to deliver the baby. Alternatively, if she does not reach full dilation, or if the baby becomes further distressed, a Caesarean section is performed.

The mother is groggy from the drugs and in pain from the episiotomy (or the Caesarean). Her baby is taken from her for routine testing, but she is too drugged and tired to care. She finds it difficult to hold or nurse her child until the drugs wear off, and her newborn finds it difficult to suckle since he too is suffering from the ill-effects of the pethidine, the epidural, or the general anaesthetic.

This woman's self-confidence and self-esteem are diminished. She feels cheated, and that her body has let her down. She has no sense of power and achievement. She feels that she has been violated, and resents the baby for causing her so much pain and distress. She also feels quite detached from him and is happy to let him be taken to the nursery while she sleeps off the effects of the drugs.

When she wakes she feels miserable. This definitely isn't how she thought it would be. She knows that something is very wrong but is unable to say exactly what it is. Her baby is brought to her and she feels nothing. She cries, but consoles herself that lots of women suffer from 'baby blues' and all the books assure her that, in time, she will come to love her newborn.

We know this second account, or something very like it, is the story of countless women. Today, '*A mother giving birth*' is the story of a small minority of very fortunate women. (Janette can remember one of the first Nursing Mothers' meetings she ever attended. The new mothers were discussing their baby's birth and the days and weeks following the birth. With one exception (that being Jan) they had all been '*A woman delivered of her baby*.') Despite some very positive changes occurring in birthing practices, the majority of women still experience the birth of their child as a surgically assisted procedure, rather than a spontaneous act of bringing forth new life.

But a labour and birth are generally over in a very short space of time (generally less than 24 hours). Does it really matter if your birth is a surgical operation or not? Surely any adverse effects will be minimal and short-lived? If these sentiments are a reflection of your thinking, let's look closely at the benefits that a natural birth bestows on a new family.

ADVANTAGES OF AN ACTIVE NATURAL BIRTH

Your body is ready

When you go into spontaneous labour at full term your body and your baby are both ready. The hormone relaxin has prepared muscles and ligaments for giving birth. The copper levels, which have risen steadily during the latter stages of your pregnancy, have caused zinc to pack into the placenta. These high copper levels may act as a trigger for the initiation of labour.

During a normal, unmedicated labour, your body produces endorphins. These are morphine-like substances that induce a sense of wellbeing and give you some protection from the pain of the contractions. If you are in a familiar environment, amongst familiar people, you will feel safe, comfortable and, hopefully, uninhibited (that's why we suggest you choose your support people carefully). All of these factors have a bearing on ensuring that uterine contractions are strong and effective. If you have some prior knowledge of what happens in each stage of labour, you will understand what is happening to your body, you will recognise the strength and power of the whole process and be free to work with it rather than resist it.

You will expedite the labour and birth

When you are free to move around you will intuitively adopt the positions that feel most comfortable: kneeling, standing, squatting and sitting. These positions have one thing in common—the birth canal is vertical (rather than horizontal) which means you have the assistance of gravity when giving birth to your baby. Numerous scientific studies have confirmed what women have known for thousands of years: an upright position has many advantages, as listed below, over a horizontal position for giving birth.

Advantages of being upright and active
- The uterine contractions are more effective.
- The uterine contractions are more regular.
- The dilation of the cervix is greater.
- Relaxation between contractions is more complete.
- Both first and second stages of labour are shorter (up to 40 per cent shorter—yes, that's close to halving the length of your labour.)
- Less pain is experienced.

Women will usually try three or more different positions during labour. But it's important to practise in advance the stretching exercises which we recommend in Chapter 5, since some of the positions which are most helpful for relieving pain, and for facilitating the birth, might be uncomfortable at first.

You will be in control
If your support people are able to offer the comfort of massage and hot packs, and if you can enjoy a warm bath or shower, you won't find the pain of the contractions completely overwhelming. If you are able to drink freely you won't become dehydrated. You might need to eat as well, and small frequent snacks of complex carbohydrates provide your body with a constant supply of glucose.

If you labour at your own pace, in sympathetic surroundings, you really need little more than appropriate encouragement, physical contact and comfort. If your midwife is there to support you physically and emotionally while she just watches and waits, you will be much less likely to sustain any trauma to your body.

You will be fulfilled and empowered
The pain of childbirth can be thought of symbolically, as a challenge that a woman must overcome, or an initiation through which she must pass, to become a mother. To do this successfully, she must draw on inner resources that she may never have drawn on before, or which she may not even have realised she possessed.

But in passing through this initiation, a woman feels totally empowered. This feeling of power, and a strong sense of belief in self, gives her a very firm base from which she is best able to cope with the challenges of mothering that lie ahead. Also, the trust she has gained in her body and her firm belief in the rightness of letting nature take its course, will serve her well for following a natural path through feeding and nurturing her baby and parenting her children.

If you actively and consciously give birth to your baby you will be full of a sense of achievement which will lead to a vastly improved interaction with your newborn. If you are able to nurse your baby immediately after birth you will have little difficulty in establishing breastfeeding. You will find that this early breastfeeding causes your uterus to contract rapidly, which reduces the risk of bleeding or postpartum haemorrhage. You will also find that nursing your baby straight away enhances the bonding process and heightens your feelings of fulfilment.

Your baby is ready

There are lots of benefits for you, but lots of ways in which your baby will benefit from a completely natural birth too. He prepares himself for labour by producing stress hormones so that at birth he is primed to breathe and survive independently, so it's important that he is allowed to come when he's ready. After a natural, spontaneous labour and birth he will be aware that he entered the world at his own pace and without unnecessary interference. We now know that a baby in the womb is capable of feeling and sensing a great deal. Even though his birth experience is something which he will not consciously remember, there are indications that babies who have been induced may carry a life-long memory pattern of their induction, which can result in their feeling constantly rushed or hurried.

When labour begins, your baby is usually in a head down position. This doesn't just happen. A healthy baby who is ready to be born is very much part of the process, not just an inert passenger. He is an integral part of your labour and will actually wriggle into the optimum position for passing down the birth canal, bracing himself against the top of your uterus to do so. His head presses down and this (his own weight) and his vertical position help your cervix to open. However, these normal, helpful responses will be dulled by any drugs that you might be given.

Your baby will be relaxed but alert

After a labour without drugs, or intervention of any sort, and born away from cold, noise and lights, your baby will be relaxed but alert. If you place him immediately on your belly or breast, and stroke and touch him, the important process of bonding can take place to best advantage. If your baby's umbilical cord is allowed to stop pulsing before it is cut, this will ensure his breathing is well established. If he is not separated from you and if he is allowed to breastfeed just as soon as he needs to, then he will feel that the world into which he has come is a safe and caring place.

The whole family will bond

From the moment of birth all the family members who are present have a connection with one another. Your partner has a strong and immediate bond with his child as well as a deepened respect for you when he sees how hard you have worked. For siblings, their anxiety at the arrival of a new baby can be overcome if they do not feel isolated from the birth.

A profound experience

But ultimately, giving birth as nature intended is a profound experience. It is difficult and challenging, yet rewarding and enriching. It is an awe-inspiring event from which you should be able to draw strength and power all your life. Sheila Kitzinger has this to say: '*To carry a child in your body, to plan ahead, to make choices between alternatives, to give birth and hold your child in your arms is an experience that can bring with it profound emotional commitment, deep acceptance of responsibility, and a maturing of personality. It is not a medical event. It is a major life transition!*'

DISADVANTAGES OF MEDICAL MANAGEMENT

What then, of a medically managed delivery? We'll now consider all the interventions or medical procedures that make up the practice of interventionist obstetrics. We'll look at the reasons that might be given for performing these procedures. We'll discuss whether these reasons are valid (and, therefore, whether the procedures are actually necessary). Finally, we'll tell you what adverse effects they may have on you and your baby.

Birth 'options'—true options?

Over the last 50 years the medical profession has convinced women that they cannot give birth without medical help, and that if they labour without all the latest technology close at hand, they risk both their life and the life of their child as well. Today, the majority of women in Australia give birth in a hospital, when only 60 or 70 years ago they gave birth to their babies at home.

Birthing women are confronted by numerous medical procedures that are often casually referred to as 'options'. However an option indicates freedom to choose, or at least a choice which will lead to an equal outcome, so in most instances these procedures are not true options at all. Usually they are offered when you are not in a position to make a completely rational and informed decision. *'Just to help things along'* or *'for your safety'*, or for the *'wellbeing of your baby'* are emotive and seductive inducements. It is a rare labouring woman who can resist a little bit of assistance, or make the choice which she has been told by the apparent experts might put herself or her baby in jeopardy.

Despite assurances that the procedures are in your best interests, they may have side effects, they may be stressful, they may lead to further medical intervention, or to surgical procedures, and ultimately they may interfere with the bonding process. In other words they have the potential to adversely affect your physical, mental and emotional health and the health of your newborn. What is more, their use may have been completely unnecessary in the first place.

In 1989, an Australian Government publication, *National Women's Health Policy—Advancing Women's Health in Australia*, had this to say: *It is highly questionable whether as many women would consent to surgical intervention (induction, forceps, Caesarean sections) if they were aware of the potential risks to the mother of infection, maternal incontinence and death. Risks to the child include nerve injuries, respiratory distress, bleeding, bruises and fractures.*

Also, a 1999 Senate committee report into birth practices in Australia, *Rocking the Cradle*, identifies that many women want more from their birth experiences than they feel they are able to experience under the present system, and recommends that they should be able to get it. The report concludes that childbirth is 'over-medicalised' and that this leads to higher levels of intervention, 'consequent morbidity, and . . . the disempowerment of women giving birth'. As well as recommendations regarding birth practices, (which we'll refer to later), it recommends restricting the use of ultrasound during pregnancy, as the medical benefits are 'unproven'.

Many disadvantages go hand in hand with all the 'options' offered by the medical model. We'll look at the general problems of stress and the side effects of intervention first before examining the impact of specific procedures on you and your baby.

Stress inhibits labour

The hormone adrenaline is secreted when your body is under stress. Adrenaline will be produced when you are in a situation where you are not entirely relaxed: if you are in an unfamiliar environment, or if you are undergoing a physical examination or other medical procedure. Since adrenaline inhibits the effects of oxytocin, which is the hormone causing your uterus to contract, stress reduces the effectiveness of your contractions considerably.

So the simple act of going to the hospital and filling in the admission forms can initiate the production of adrenaline. An internal examination to assess your progress will normally be performed when you are admitted, and this can be quite stressful (and sometimes painful as well). Adrenaline will also be produced if you are labouring in the presence of strangers. We talked earlier of the ideal place for giving birth being similar to that in which to make love—both are equally intimate acts. It's hardly surprising that you'll feel uncomfortable if the doctors and midwives around you are not familiar faces. It's certainly no coincidence that lots of women arrive at the hospital in strong labour, only to be sent home after a few hours when their labour has slowed to a halt.

Interventions disturb the natural rhythm of labour

Women come in many shapes, sizes and temperaments, and there are many lengths, intensities and paces of labours. All interventions, no matter how well intentioned, interfere with the normal and totally individual rhythm of the birthing process. Once that natural rhythm is broken or interfered with, it is almost inevitable that still further intervention will be necessary. Sheila Kitzinger refers to this effect as the cascade of intervention.

Your obstetrician's reassurance that he will intervene 'only when indicated' can also be open to a variety of interpretations. The indications can be varied to suit the circumstances, and the circumstances can be as irrelevant to your birth as whether he has a social function to attend as your labour progresses. Fewer babies are born on Sundays and public holidays than at other times of the year and births also seem to peak before holidays such as Christmas. Take a look at the hospital statistics if you're in any doubt.

The decision to intervene may also depend on whether or not your labour is conforming to the 'normal' curve when, in reality, there is no such thing as a normal labour. The variations in length, intensity and degrees of progress are endless, even for the same woman giving birth to subsequent children. This is hardly surprising when you consider that your baby has an individual temperament and he is very much an actor in this drama!

Let's look now at some of those interventions or 'options' that you might be offered. They might seem innocuous enough at first glance, or if they are considered on their own, but just remember that each one can easily, and does frequently, lead to others.

Common medical interventions

Induction
Your pregnancy will last for nine lunar months, or 266 days from the date of conception (a lunar month is approximately 29½ days). More

commonly, your due date is calculated as 40 weeks following the first day of your last menstrual period. But just as women have menstrual cycles of varying lengths, just as children grow at different rates, just as each one of us is physically different, babies grow in utero at varying rates too. Be assured that an absolutely normal pregnancy can last anywhere from 38 to 42 weeks. In other words, two weeks either side of the estimated due date of 40 weeks is within completely accept-able limits and 10 per cent of pregnancies proceed beyond 42 weeks.

However, though many doctors consider an induction necessary once a woman is past her due date, if the placenta is functioning ade-quately you can be confident that your baby will be born when he is good and ready. Studies have shown that induction for post-maturity does not improve the eventual outcome and increases the Caesarean section rate by as much as five times. It seems that vigilant non-intervention up to the forty-fourth week does not jeopardise either mother or baby.

Furthermore, the size and growth of a baby are not the same thing and individual babies all have their own pattern as we have already explained. This individual pattern may depend on factors such as maternal nutrition, genetics and ethnicity. The practice of inducing a baby diagnosed as suffering from foetal growth retardation (FGR) is highly questionable anyway, since the uterine environment is simply replaced with the dubious option of a humidicrib. If you are faced with an induction, a cardiotocograph (CTG) can reassure you that all is well. Keeping a simple kick chart (see Chapter 9), which really allows you to tune into your baby's movements, can also be useful.

Sometimes, due to a condition such as toxaemia (which can threaten your safety and that of your baby), an induction will be medically necessary. However, an induction is never justified simply because you are tired of waiting or because you have had a certain birth date in your mind for the last nine months. Nor should an induc-tion ever be scheduled for your obstetrician's convenience. The most popular method of induction (or augmentation) uses syntocinon, a synthetic hormone that mimics the action of oxytocin, the hormone which is naturally produced by your body and which causes your uterus to contract. This natural production of oxytocin is perfectly tailored to meet your needs. It ensures that the intensity of the con-tractions increases gradually, which allows you time to become accustomed to the pain and to be able to deal with it adequately.

However, administration of the synthetic product is unlikely to produce such finely tuned results. It may fail to have an effect at all, or conversely, it may cause extremely powerful contractions that occur back to back, with no interval between them. If you have no time to gather your energy and your mental resources between contractions, or if the pain is suddenly of great intensity, you will inevitably request pain relief.

Augmentation

Augmentation (using syntocinon) may be ordered if your own contractions diminish in strength or intensity, or if dilation is slow. This can occur when your body produces the stress hormone adrenaline. If you feel apprehensive or uneasy in any way (which is not unlikely in a hospital full of strange faces, routines and equipment), the adrenaline that is produced will inhibit the effect of oxytocin, the strength of your contractions will be reduced and the progress of your labour will slow. The syntocinon may help, but, as with its use in induction, may fail to have an effect or may produce overwhelmingly strong and frequent contractions.

Other methods of induction and augmentation include artificial rupture of the membranes (ARM) and the use of prostaglandin gels. However, like the use of syntocinon, neither of these methods can really duplicate the complex set of factors that spontaneously initiate and maintain labour.

Drugs

Other drugs that are commonly used in labour may adversely affect you and your baby in a number of ways. You may wish to be informed of these effects before deciding whether to use them.

Antibiotics

Those of you who are booked into hospital for your birth will probably have a vaginal swab taken at 28 weeks to test for Strep B infection. Between five per cent and 30 per cent of women will test positive, even though there may be no symptoms. There is concern, however, about the effects on the newborn baby such as generalised infection, breathing difficulties, pneumonia and rheumatic fever. Transmission usually occurs during labour, especially after the waters have broken (though there is no risk during pregnancy of infection, it can contribute to a premature birth). However, this risk is very small (about 0.01 per cent) and is more likely to affect premature babies.

Despite this small risk, most hospitals have a program of intravenous antibiotics to be administered during labour. While we recommend diagnosis and treatment of Strep B in the preconception period, we are not so convinced of the benefits of IV antibiotics given during birth, as it's possible that the antibiotics will have a negative effect on your baby's intestinal flora, which are required, amongst other important considerations, for the absorption of nutrients and the production of vitamin K (see Chapter 10).

Drugs for premature births

If your baby is very early, there may be an attempt to stall the contractions through the use of drugs which relax the uterine muscle, but studies have questioned not only their safety, but their effectiveness. Corticosteroid drugs are also routinely administered to help the foetal lungs to mature. If your baby is then placed in an incubator (this depends on his size and condition) drugs may continue to be administered until his development is such that survival is ensured.

Drugs for induction and pain relief

The release of endorphins—the morphine-like, natural painkillers that are manufactured by your body—can be inhibited by the drugs used to induce labour and also by drugs that are given for pain relief. These same drugs can also adversely affect the production of oxytocin. Consequently, painkilling drugs not only reduce levels of naturally produced analgesic substances, but they hinder your labour's normal progress. As well, narcotic analgesics (such as pethidine) can greatly alter your perception and diminish your ability to participate actively in the birth.

Drugs can also inhibit the release of the very important stress hormones that are produced by your baby's body to prepare him for his existence outside the womb. Drugs of the narcotic variety will affect his perception as well as yours and he may not attach to the nipple or be able to breastfeed successfully. These drugs also have the ability to cause respiratory depression, and any drug will be an excessive load for his immature system to metabolise and excrete.

The drugs that are used for general or epidural anaesthesia initiate massive free radical damage and dramatically increase your body's needs for all the antioxidant nutrients such as vitamins A, C and E, zinc and selenium for at least six weeks after the birth.

Epidural anaesthetics

An epidural anaesthetic is a popular method of pain relief which is frequently suggested for:

- long labours (if the baby is in a posterior position).
- breech presentation (as they reduce the urge to push, when the cervix is not fully dilated).
- high forceps delivery, which may also be used if your baby needs turning.
- if pre-eclampsia or high blood pressure is a problem during labour.
- for a Caesarean section.

Epidurals leave you mentally alert, but they block all sensation in your lower body. This ensures that you feel no pain from the contractions, but you will also have little knowledge of how your labour is progressing. Once an epidural is administered you will no longer be able to move around but will be confined to a horizontal position, which is a physiologically unsound one for a woman giving birth. In this position you are no longer working with your body or with gravity. It has been estimated that the opening of the birth canal is reduced by 25–30 per cent if you remain horizontal, so the downward journey of your baby is significantly hindered. There are other disadvantages of a supine, passive labour, as outlined below. (It is possible, in some hospitals, to have a 'mobile epidural', so you can still move and walk around.)

When administered skilfully, an epidural may be timed to wear off as you approach the end of the first stage of labour. This allows the return of sensation to the lower half of your body and allows you to actively participate in the second stage. In other words you will have the experience of pushing your baby out. However, exact timing of this degree means having an extremely skilled anaesthetist, one who is able to judge your progress accurately. Unfortunately, this level of skill isn't always present, and furthermore, the procedure is not free of side effects. These include infection, severe headaches, temporary paralysis and long-term back problems. An epidural anaesthetic can cross the placenta, adversely affecting your baby. Maternal blood pressure may be lowered, thereby reducing the blood flow to the placenta, which has the potential to cause further harm to your baby.

The 1999 Senate committee report, *Rocking the Cradle*, noted that the incidence of epidurals was increasing, and warned of the cascade of intervention that could follow, including greater use of forceps, vacuum extraction and Caesareans.

A supine, passive labour

As well as defying gravity and fighting your baby's descent, lying on your back can trigger complications.

- It compresses the descending aorta, which can lead to foetal distress.
- It compresses the inferior vena cava, which can contribute to maternal hypertension and haemorrhage.
- It negates the mobility of your pelvic bones and the flexibility of your pelvic muscles.
- It causes your perineum to stretch unevenly so it's more likely that an episiotomy will be required.

The disadvantages of giving birth passively are summed up by three experts:

'Except for being hanged by the feet, the supine position is the worst conceivable position for labour and delivery' —Dr Caldeyro-Barcia, International Federation of Gynaecologists and Obstetricians

'No animal species adopts such a disadvantageous position during such an important and critical event' —Dr Peter Dunn, Consultant Senior Lecturer in Child Health, Southmead Hospital, Bristol

'All over the world and throughout recorded history women have chosen upright positions to give birth and it is only we in the West who have had the extraordinary notion that a woman should lie on her back with her legs in the air to deliver a baby' —Sheila Kitzinger, birth-educator, activist, author and mother

Lack of nourishment

The energy that you will use up during labour has been compared to that expended during a brisk 6-kilometre hike. Yet some maternity units allow you no food or drink once you've been admitted. This strict cautionary measure is designed to ensure that you inhale no vomit should you need to be anaesthetised prior to undergoing a Caesarean section. However, there are no studies to show that a properly anaesthetised woman will inhale her own vomit, and this measure denies nourishment to the 80 per cent of women who do not undergo a Caesarean section.

You need energy and water while you're in labour, and while you may not be in need of a three-course meal, small nutritious snacks and appropriate fluid intake are essential if your labour is not to lead to dehydration and depleted glucose levels. If your glucose levels fall, as they may in the case of a longer labour during which you receive no nourishment, you will develop a condition called ketosis. This occurs when your muscles can no longer obtain sufficient glucose for their proper contraction and start to burn fat as fuel. It indicates that your muscles are exhausted and are no longer capable of working properly.

Dextrose drips are designed to prevent this condition, but they have several disadvantages. With a drip in your arm you are unable to be fully active and will almost certainly be confined to bed. As well, this elevated concentration of a simple carbohydrate can cause hyperglycaemia (high blood sugar levels) in your baby. These high blood sugar levels will fall to well below normal after birth (hypoglycaemia). Since your baby's body depends on a constant and stable supply of blood sugar to maintain all its functions, these fluctuating levels can have serious implications for a newborn's ability to adapt to life outside the womb. The same fluctuations can leave you feeling both physically and mentally debilitated.

Foetal monitoring

Foetal monitoring, which was originally designed for use in high-risk labours, has now become almost routine procedure. In some labour wards it seems to have taken the place of the comfort, support, and careful observation which was once offered by midwives. Your baby's heartbeat may be monitored indirectly by an electronic device strapped to your abdomen, or directly by attaching an electrode to the baby's scalp via your vagina. The second method is obviously extremely stressful for your baby and for you as well.

The readout from the monitor has great potential for misinterpretation, with the accuracy depending on the experience and skill of the technician. An incorrect diagnosis of distress can result in unnecessary surgical intervention. Misinterpretation aside, both monitoring methods interfere with your ability to move around and to change position. Consequently, being attached to a monitor of either type will adversely affect your ability to deal with the pain of the contractions, and assuming a horizontal position will slow the progress of your labour as we've already described.

Episiotomy

An episiotomy will usually be necessary to help the baby out if you've had any (or all) of the foregoing procedures. An episiotomy is a straight cut through both muscle and connective tissue to enlarge the opening of the vagina. It is quite unlike a tear, which may be ragged, but which is largely superficial. It is frequently performed without anaesthesia, when the pressure of the baby's head on your perineum is considered to have deadened all feeling in the area. Such an incision is not only very stressful but extremely painful as well, and certainly more painful than tearing. Many women suffer long-term discomfort (particularly during sexual intercourse) and incontinence after undergoing an episiotomy and its repair.

In 1985 The World Health Organisation (WHO) issued a statement saying that the 'systematic use of episiotomy is not justified' and followed that in 1992 by claiming that it 'should be abandoned'.

Despite this, in Australia, the episiotomy rate varies greatly from hospital to hospital, reaching a peak of almost 40 per cent at hospitals in the higher socio-economic area of Sydney, to a low and much more acceptable two per cent in a few small country hospitals. The overall rate is 20 per cent for *all* women (1996 statistics). While it is possible that the higher rates for all forms of intervention at large metropolitan teaching hospitals reflect the numbers of high-risk pregnancies and births which are transferred there, the episiotomy rate for births occurring at home is virtually zero.

Delivery by forceps

For centuries, forceps were the only medical interventions available to a woman whose labour was not progressing well. These days, if the wellbeing of a mother or baby is considered to be threatened, it's more likely that a Caesarean section will be recommended. However, forceps are still used if the labour is in second stage, the cervix fully dilated, the membranes have ruptured and the baby's head has fully engaged and descended to a certain degree but fails to come down any further, or if baby or mother become distressed at this stage.

Obstetrical forceps are applied to either side of the baby's head. The pressure which is applied during a forceps delivery is considerable and may result in bruising, fractures, nerve damage and neck or spine dislocation. Chiropractors and osteopaths, who specialise in cranio-sacral therapy, are now recognising many serious and long-term ill effects, including learning problems, that can be a result of this type of surgical delivery. The mother may also suffer problems including perineal, cervical and vaginal tears, urinary and faecal incontinence, prolapse and long-term pain. Sometimes forceps are used (with an episiotomy) for premature babies to protect their softer skulls from the pressure of the birth canal.

Vacuum extraction

Vacuum extraction (or ventouse) is an alternative method that may be used to pull your baby from your body. This method, which involves the use of a pump, will severely distort your baby's head at the site where the suction cap is applied.

Caesarean section

A Caesarean section is the most invasive of all the interventionist procedures. It is major surgery and with it go all the attendant risks. Mothers who have undergone this procedure also appear more likely to suffer from postnatal depression and take longer to recover from the birth. A Caesarean involves a longer stay in hospital for both mother and baby, with a higher risk of infection. Further vaginal deliveries may be compromised, though this risk is often over-stated. Paradoxi-cally, since Caesareans are commonly performed to avoid problems, or in some cases to protect the doctor against a lawsuit, there's a much higher risk of complications than with a vaginal birth. Even repeat Caesareans carry a greater risk than a subsequent vaginal birth. Haemorrhage is six times more likely, the mother has five times the risk of death and there may be complications due to anaesthesia. The baby also faces greater risks, including a higher risk of neonatal death, jaundice, respiratory distress and all the problems associated with anaesthesia. Apart from these risks, it has also been found that the baby born by Caesarean section is disadvantaged in a number of other ways, due to the fact that the child born by this method has fewer stress hormones and has received little or none of the stimulation of a normal vaginal birth. Studies show that these babies reach developmental milestones behind their peers. Bonding is disturbed, breastfeeding may be difficult to establish (because of the pain), and grieving over the loss of the birth experience may last for months or years.

Some women choose an elective Caesarean so that they can schedule their child's birth to fit in with a busy career or other schedule, or simply to avoid the pain of labour (though the postoperative pain of a Caesarean will be debilitating and longer lasting). Others may undergo a Caesarean for their obstetrician's convenience. Caesareans are frequently ordered for a multiple birth, if the baby is in a breech position, or for the spurious condition which is termed cephalo-pelvic disproportion (when your baby's head is supposedly too big for your pelvic outlet). Other women, who have had a Caesarean previously, are persuaded by the erroneous belief that 'once a Caesarean, always a Caesarean'. Finally, many women undergo a Caesarean simply because they are victims of the cascade of obstetrical interventions which we have just described. However, none of these are valid reasons for performing a procedure that should be reserved for genuine medical emergencies. Such emergencies are far fewer in number than you might think and again hospital statistics are enlightening. In Sydney, the Caesarean section rate reaches 30 per cent in the same hospitals which boast the highest episiotomy rates, yet falls to one-third of this in some country hospitals. This is the rate (10–15 per cent) which the World Health Organisation recommends should not be exceeded in any geographical area. Overall, Australia's rate is assessed at around 20 per cent with a higher rate occurring amongst privately insured patients, those giving birth in major tertiary hospitals and those attended by specialist obstetricians. These differences are not fully explained by the greater proportion of older and high-risk women in these groups. This was noted in the Senate committee report, *Rocking the Cradle*, (mentioned previously), when reporting the current Caesarean rate in Australia, with which it was particularly concerned. The report found that too many medically unjustified surgical interventions were being performed and proposed that a rate of 15 per cent was appropriate, and that attempts should be made to achieve this.

The potential for birth trauma

Babies who have been traumatised during the birth process (by the use of forceps, for example) have a greater tendency to left–right brain dysfunction. This may manifest as dyslexia, learning problems or lack of co-ordination. (Of course, babies born naturally may also suffer birth trauma.) Treatments for birth trauma can be found in Chapter 12. Rebirthing, where the trauma of birthing is re-experienced and transformed through breathing techniques, has been used to help adults overcome some of the emotional consequences of a traumatic birth.

Your sense of power and achievement will be diminished

Despite everything we've just said, obstetrical interventions have saved the lives of countless mothers and their babies. But many labours, which should progress to normal, uncomplicated vaginal births, become surgically assisted deliveries because of the cascade effect of interventionist procedures. Even though a procedure might be performed with the very best of intentions, it invariably leads to further intervention and we showed how this can easily happen in the story of 'A woman is delivered of her baby', page 23.

Apart from the many side effects of the various procedures and the considerable levels of stress to which you and your baby may be subjected, any intervention will interfere with the way in which you perceive your birth. It will determine whether you see it as a uniquely empowering experience, or one in which you feel cheated and disempowered.

The type of birth you and your baby experience will affect the way in which you nurture him in those critically important early hours and days. Nature has designed an extraordinarily effective system to ensure that a newborn infant is loved, protected, cared for and nurtured adequately, and this system operates most effectively when you experience a completely natural birth and when the exquisitely sensitive period of bonding, which follows, unfolds without interruption. While many of the ill effects of a poor birth experience can be overcome, you and your baby are off to a flying start in your life together if you have been able to experience a better birth and better bonding. This early bonding establishes a pattern that will have consequences for the rest of your child's life. It will have effects on his relationship with both you and your partner, as well as with his brothers and sisters. It will affect how he perceives himself and his immediate environment and how he eventually relates to the wider community and to the world at large. A 'better birth' and 'better bonding' have benefits that extend well beyond those few momentous hours in which both take place.

Choosing
your team

Now you know what (mostly) happens during labour and birth, and have seen the vast differences in the way women may experience them, you'll need to choose the people you want to support you through your special time. As well as a professional carer, think about who else you'll want and need to be present to make your birth 'better'.

YOUR CARER

Although it's not necessary to rush off the moment you've conceived and put yourself in the care of a professional, it may be wise to give some thought early on to the carers you would prefer to support you through the pregnancy and birth. For example, as midwives are in scant supply, some get booked up well in advance.

Obstetric care

We have described the medical management of labour and birth, but we don't want you to think that all obstetricians are stuck in the medical mindset. Many realise that birth is a momentous event and will make every effort to allow women to experience it fully, without intervention. They are aware that a woman's desire to actively participate in the birth of her baby, rather than adopt the role of passive patient, is absolutely valid and must be honoured. Female obstetricians may fall into this category more frequently than males, since they have often given birth themselves, and this may influence your choice of carer.

If you decide on obstetric care, it's good if you have a personal referral from someone who had expectations that were similar to your own, and who found that their obstetrician respected their wishes. If you don't have any close friends who have given birth recently, make some inquiries before you make a decision. Doctors who are registered with birthing centres are likely to be more sympathetic to a natural and non-interventionist approach, but it's good to keep the following facts in mind.

- Obstetricians are trained to 'manage' pregnancy, labour and birth.

- Their experience is, almost without exception, of labours that have been induced, augmented and monitored.

- They are skilled in performing episiotomies, forceps deliveries and Caesarean sections.

- They invariably associate labour with strong pain that must be relieved.

- They may have little experience of spontaneous labours that result in a vaginal delivery without some form of intervention.

- They are often unaware of the enormous variations in individual labours.

- They may set completely arbitrary time limits, which mean that you are labouring against the clock.

- Their focus is on the physical side of birth, and they are often insensitive to its profound emotional and spiritual aspects.

Midwifery care

If you choose midwifery care, then you alone are responsible for your baby's birth, and your attendants will do little more than watch, wait and support. You and your baby are also viewed as an integral unit and if the needs of one are met, so are the needs of the other. Midwifery care is holistic care. The following facts are also important to remember.

- 'Midwife' means 'with woman'.

- Midwives have always been the traditional attendants and carers at births.

- The training of midwives has quite a different perspective to that of medical specialists.

- Although midwives are well trained in all the medical aspects of birth and are able to manage emergencies capably and quickly, their role is that of facilitator and care giver.

- They are present to offer guidance and emotional support.

- They may do little more than observe and wait, offering physical comfort such as massage, words of encouragement, and, occasionally, advice.

- They are instinctive, intuitive and empathetic.

- Most have given birth themselves.

- Their role is not to intervene, but their skills are such that they can determine if and when intervention is necessary.

- Statistics clearly show that there are fewer interventions and perinatal mortality rates are much lower when births take place with only a midwife in attendance.

- Some hospitals now have midwifery clinics which allow women to choose midwives as their primary carers but still provide access to obstetric care if necessary.

Before you make your decision about whether you want obstetric or midwifery care, a look at the hospital statistics which relate to intervention rates can be very informative. These figures are usually compiled annually and will be available from your state health department. For example, NSW data is published in a booklet called *Public Health Bulletin Supplement—New South Wales Mothers and Babies.*

You can see at a glance which hospitals have the highest (and the lowest) rates of induction, epidurals, episiotomies and Caesareans. From these figures you will see that some of the procedures are still almost routine in some maternity units, and knowing this, you can make a much more informed decision about where, and with whom, you would like to give birth to your baby.

Some of the statistics will inevitably reflect the fact that the teaching hospitals in large cities receive many pregnancy complications and transfers from smaller regional or country hospitals. Consequently, the intervention rates for these large institutions will reflect this to some extent. However, Dr Marsden Wagner, an epidemiologist with the World Health Organisation, has shown that the higher rate of interventions in large teaching hospitals is out of proportion with the number of high risk births and pregnancies, including transfers. It is possible that the specialists who practise at these hospitals may be inclined to view all labours and births as complicated, since they see a preponderance of those that are.

You may also find the World Health Organisation's 1985 recommendations for appropriate technology at birth, which we set out here, useful in reaching your decision.

※ There should be self-care in the period around the time of the birth.

※ Women's mutual aid groups should be available to offer support and information. This would enable women to choose the type of birth they prefer.

※ Induction should be reserved for specific indications, and no geographic region should have induction rates greater than 10 per cent.

※ Artificial early rupture of the membranes is not scientifically justified.

※ Women should not be put in a lithotomy position. They should be free to move and the individual woman should decide the position in which to deliver.

⚬ There is no evidence that electronic foetal monitoring (EFM) has any positive effect on the outcome of pregnancy. EFM should be carried out only in carefully selected medical cases.

⚬ The routine administration of analgesic or anaesthetic drugs should be avoided.

⚬ The systematic use of episiotomy is not justified.

⚬ There is no justification for any geographic area to have a rate for Caesarean sections that is greater than 10–15 per cent.

⚬ The team caring for the mother and child before, during and after the birth should be motivated to enhance relationships between mother, child and family.

⚬ Observation of a healthy newborn does not justify separation from his mother.

⚬ Following the birth, there should be immediate beginning of breastfeeding before the mother leaves the delivery room.

Whether you decide to be cared for by an obstetrician or a midwife, together with your partner you should agree on what you want and what you wish to avoid and make your wishes clear to your carer. You must ask for your desires and hopes for your birth to be written on your medical records. You should also prepare a birth plan and we'll give you some suggestions in Chapter 8.

THE FATHER

Women have always been the traditional attendants at births, although in some communities the husband underwent a mock labour while his wife was undergoing the real thing. However, he was almost never present for the birth, and women friends and relatives filled most of the roles that, today, are filled by a husband or partner. These women were extended family, or they were friends and confidantes. They helped with all sorts of child-raising and household tasks, so it was logical for them to support the labouring woman in something considered strictly women's business.

When birth moved to the province of the hospital, men were still unwelcome visitors, consigned to pacing the hospital corridors, or to smoking cigarettes and drinking beer in the company of their mates, while waiting for the phone call to announce their baby's arrival. There is no doubt that some suffered a sense of exclusion. Janette's father remembers standing on an orange crate outside a hospital window to see his wife and newborn daughter. In the 1940s and '50s, most fathers glimpsed their infant only briefly through the nursery window following the birth. Francesca's father, since she was born at home in England, was confined to boiling water and ripping up sheets.

More recently, as men have taken the place of women from the extended family and have become more than just lovers and providers, they have also been welcomed into the secrets of this female business. Now the man who does not attend his child's birth is considered a bit of an oddity. But the roles of most men have changed dramatically in other ways.

Your partner may have prepared for the conception of your child with as much care as you did. (We certainly hope so.) He has probably encouraged and supported you throughout your pregnancy and may have adhered to the same healthy diet, exercise program and lifestyle changes as you. (Ditto.) He will have been involved in learning about the growth of your baby in the uterus, he has been a party to the decisions about antenatal testing and about other choices concerning where, with whom, and how your baby is to make his entrance into the world. (Well done, Dad!) Together you attended childbirth education classes (see Chapter 6), and now the logical extension of all this interest and involvement is his role as support person during your labour.

The bonds between parent and child which are established after your baby is born are as important for the father as they are for the mother. Witnessing the birth of his child is an extraordinarily powerful emotional experience for a man and it sets the scene for continuing involvement and support throughout your child's life. If you have this sort of support from your partner, you are off to a wonderful start. The feeling of intimacy and sharing which you establish means he won't feel alienated or excluded in those early months when your baby takes an enormous amount of your love, attention and time.

His support during your labour may take the form of massage, stroking, back rubbing, application of hot packs or towels and carefully chosen words of encouragement. He can help when you want to change position, embrace you, physically support you, and may even be able to catch the baby and later, cut the umbilical cord. He may also need to act as an advocate for non-intervention if you think you can't continue and are ready to ask for pain relief. Sometimes just a few words to tell you how well you're doing are all that is needed. He can also act as an ally when your attention is totally focused on what your body is doing, and you're unaware of your surroundings and other attendants. He might also be on the receiving end of some curses or curt remarks, but those childbirth education classes will have prepared him for that eventuality. But even though your partner can be an invaluable asset when you're in labour, you might want to consider having some other support people present as well.

SUPPORT PEOPLE

The best advice we can give you about support people, other than your husband or partner, is this: your baby's birth isn't a circus or a side show. Don't invite anyone simply because they've expressed a desire to be present. This experience is at least as intimate as the act of making love, so only choose someone with whom you feel absolutely comfortable and with whom you can be totally uninhibited. Clearly, this will narrow the field of potential attendees considerably. Then you should only consider those who can be completely positive and supportive. Remember that positive support is not the same as sympathy. You don't want someone (e.g. your mother) saying, 'I hate to see you in so much pain.' You need encouragement and a few carefully chosen words about your progress.

If there's nobody in your circle of family or friends who really fills the bill, then you might be wise to have only your partner and your midwife in attendance. If you've chosen obstetric care, just remember that if all is going well it's likely that your doctor will only look in briefly, or turn up at the last minute, though the hospital midwives will be dropping in and out.

If you'd really like another support person, then your childbirth educator might be able to put you in touch with someone who acts in the manner of a trained *doula*. 'Doula' is a Greek word that is translated as 'woman's servant', and though this person might be professionally trained to offer guidance, encouragement, advice and any explanations which might be necessary, she does not perform any clinical tasks. Numerous studies show that women who labour in the presence of constant support have shorter labours and fewer interventions. So if you're going to a hospital or birthing centre and want to be absolutely certain that you will have someone with you at all times, finding an appropriately trained support person is a worthwhile endeavour. In a birthing centre there will be attendant midwives, and you will be able to include your own independent midwife if she is accredited at the centre. However, in a labour ward she will be able to do little but stand by and offer support, as she will not be permitted to take part in any medical procedures.

If you're uncertain about your life partner's ability to be present at the appropriate time, look for someone else who can definitely be there for you. If you're unsure about your partner's ability to be truly helpful, or if he's really uncomfortable with the whole idea, you're better off without that sort of negative energy. In this case you might decide to revert to the idea of a traditional women-only birth.

CHILDREN AT THE BIRTH

You might be warned that young children may become distressed if they see their mother in pain during labour, but it's a fact that if they have been prepared for what to expect at a birth, children handle the whole experience with amazing equanimity. There are many good books with clear, simple illustrations that you can use to teach them about pregnancy, labour and birth (see Recommended Reading).

Small children may find the first stage of labour less than interesting. They will probably be happy to come and go, and they should be completely free to do so. Don't forget that, depending on their ages, they'll need food, drink, sleep, care, comfort, and entertainment, so it's important that there is a support person present whose role is simply to look after the children. They must feel absolutely comfortable with this person and happy to be in their care, because you definitely don't need the distraction of trying to attend to their needs while you're in labour.

If children are encouraged to touch the new baby, to kiss him and hold his hands, they will be bonded to him as soon as he is born. You may be able to avoid a lot of genuine sibling rivalry if the whole family is able to witness the birth of a brother or sister. We're not saying that children won't occasionally fight like cat and dog when they're older, but beneath the surface aggression there will be a very strong feeling of caring for one another. If the presence of children at the birth seems a bit radical (or perhaps it's just impractical), you should at least consider having them close at hand, and they should be encouraged to hold the new baby very shortly after the birth. This positive attitude and acceptance of birth as a normal, natural event will also be reflected in the way they later experience the birth of their own children.

WHERE WILL YOUR BABY BE BORN?

Often, the type of carer you choose will strongly influence where you will give birth. For instance, many obstetricians will only 'attend' you at certain hospitals to which independent midwives may be refused admittance. So before you make a final decision about where you're going to give birth, you need to be really sure of exactly what you want and of what you're likely to get in each place. It's also a good idea to be flexible about where you'll give birth—then you won't be too disappointed if the situation has to change.

Home

The majority of women who choose to give birth at home do so in the presence of a homebirth midwife, though there may be a very few obstetricians also willing to attend. If you have chosen to be attended by a midwife, she will see you in her home or clinic during your antenatal visits. She will probably visit you in your own home towards the end of your pregnancy. You will have the opportunity to get to know one another well, and establish that feeling of empathy and trust which is so important for a better birth. Some women choose to give birth at home without a midwife in attendance, although we don't really recommend this option, as you can't be completely sure that you won't require professional advice.

There is no doubt that choosing to have your baby at home will give you complete freedom to do what you please, and the best possible chance to have the birth that you desire. Home is the place where you will feel most relaxed and least inhibited. Home is where you can move around, take a bath, soak under the shower and ask for a massage. You can dress, undress, eat, drink, play music, burn incense and turn the lights off. You can invite anyone you like to join you and tell anyone you like to go away. You can moan, groan, sing, shout, swear or curse. It means you can do whatever you instinctively feel like doing, which is exactly what you will do to get your baby born most easily.

But if you think a homebirth is about peace and quiet, dim lights, candles burning and music softly playing then you may need to think again. Birth can be very noisy and not at all peaceful. Whether you're expecting to be blissed out, or whether you're ready for lots of raw energy and intensity, a birth at home should only be an option if you're absolutely comfortable with the normality of the process and have complete faith in your body's ability to give birth unaided. If there are any niggling doubts in the back of your mind (although we'd hope not after you've read our book), or if there are any complicating factors, then you'll need to look at the alternatives.

Birthing centre

Ideally, a birth centre combines the principal advantages of both home and hospital. If you choose a birth centre, you will see the birth centre midwives for your antenatal visits and the environment is close to what you would have at home. You will be free to move around, to change position, to have your chosen attendants (including your children) present and many of the midwives will be familiar with natural methods of pain relief (we'll discuss those in Chapter 7). But all the technology and the facilities of a hospital are just next door should they become necessary. This sense of a safety net is important for many women, and there is no doubt that many more women would opt for the security of such a centre if they could. Unfortunately, the availability of beds at birthing centres is limited, as are the numbers of such centres (although new, privately run clinics are opening in many areas). As well there are often strict guidelines used to determine who can give birth at these centres. Older women are often excluded, as are women whose babies are in the breech position, or those with a previous problematic birth history.

You might also consider choosing the personal care of a homebirth midwife who has visiting rights at a birth centre. Then you'll have all the advantages of one-on-one care during your pregnancy and a close and intimate relationship with your midwife, plus the comfort of being close to the hospital support system.

Hospital

If you think a 'relaxed hospital environment' is the safest option, be aware that this term is an oxymoron. The smooth functioning of hospitals depends on rules and regulations, routines and schedules, and you will be required to comply with them. You'll need to consider carefully whether you can handle the regimentation for a few days.

Maternity units in hospitals are certainly not the sterile, clinical places they once were. Great effort has gone into making them more like home. But even though hospital rooms may be attractively decorated and the equipment hidden away in special cabinets, if the bed is still the central piece of furniture, chances are that the hospital considers this the appropriate place for you to give birth.

However, hospital schedules and environments do vary a great deal. It is quite likely that if the hospital contains a birthing centre, then the labour ward will tend to be more flexible in its routines and also more sympathetic to an active birth process. This may be due not only to the osmotic effect of the ideology subscribed to at the birthing centre, but also to the vocal demands of women transferred to the labour ward from the birthing unit when problems arise. Some hospitals are also introducing a program of ongoing midwifery care throughout pregnancy and labour, though unfortunately, funding cuts are limiting the growth of such programs.

Just because you are giving birth in a hospital doesn't necessarily mean that there will be medical intervention, unless that is the reason that you have gone there. If you wish to reduce the possibility of unnecessary medical intervention, you should either have made your wishes plain to your birth attendants or, better still, have a knowledgeable person with you throughout labour and birth. This not only reduces your anxiety, but has been proven to reduce the chance of unwelcome or unnecessary procedures being adopted. In most situations you will be able to keep someone with you at all times, and preferably this is someone you know well and trust, and who themselves won't get anxious. It's also important that you feel confident enough, and able, to let someone know if they are distressing or confusing you.

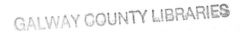

If your visit to hospital is planned, you may have had a chance to visit it and familiarise yourself with the environment, and perhaps some of the personnel, though the faces will change regularly. Even if you don't plan on ending up in a hospital, it might be useful to visit the local labour ward so you have some idea of what to expect if your plans have to change. If, or when, you go to hospital, take some familiar items with you (you could have a bag packed ready). See our suggested list in Chapter 8.

If, for medical reasons, you have no choice but hospital, you might be able to take advantage of an early discharge program. This means that if all is well you can go home soon after the birth, and will be visited daily at home by hospital midwives for up to a week. However, not all early discharges are supported by home visits, due to funding cuts. Indeed, the 1999 Senate committee report, *Rocking the Cradle*, stated that early discharges were not adequately studied before being introduced and were done as a cost-cutting exercise. The report warned that without adequate back-up, and especially if discharge occurred before breastfeeding was established, mothers could experience problems, including an increased incidence of postnatal depression.

Of course for some women a few days in hospital can seem like a holiday. If you already have children and your support group of friends and family doesn't run to help in the house after the birth, you might decide to run the gamut of the hospital routines. You might find they provide a haven of sanity and a break from thinking about kids, meals, washing, ironing, shopping and cleaning as well as your new baby.

Birth in water

If you're convinced of the benefits to your baby of the easy transition from the watery environment of the uterus to the body temperature, liquid environment of a birthing pool, then you might actually decide to give birth to your baby under water. If that is your choice, no doubt you'll do plenty of research about those benefits and about exactly what happens after your baby is born. Birthing pools may be hired and many birth centres (and some hospitals) incorporate them in their units, since immersion in water can help you relax through the pain of contractions and shorten the length of the first stage (see Chapter 7 for more on this).

We're not so sure about other perceived benefits, since your baby must still make that transition from the watery environment of the amniotic sac to the airy, terrestrial environment sooner or later. It's also interesting that some women who have chosen a water birth actually find they feel more comfortable with their feet on the ground to push their baby out. On the other hand, some women find the water such a comforting environment that, having sought it for pain relief, they actually stay in the pool or bath to give birth. Again, just go with the flow and do exactly what feels right for you. That will be right for your baby too.

Ultimately, where you give birth is not really the issue. With whom you give birth is actually much more important. It is possible to have a completely natural birth in a traditional labour ward if your attendants and carers are aware of, and sympathetic to, your desires to avoid any sort of intervention. At the end of the day, the responsibility for a better birth and better bonding rests entirely in your own hands.

Nutrition for a better birth

Like a 'better pregnancy' and a 'better baby, ' a 'better birth' has its foundations in the months before you conceive. But don't despair if it's too late for that. We're not saying that we've got an absolutely fool-proof method for ensuring that you'll be a woman who 'gives birth' if your pregnancy is already well advanced. However, there are still lots of simple, helpful things you can do to ensure that you won't be like the woman 'delivered of her baby' (see the stories in Chapter 2).

After reading about the inappropriate medical management of the birth process, you might think that the best way to ensure a 'better birth' is to have your baby at home. But, in reality, one of the most important things you can attend to is your nutritional status. If you hope to have a birth like the woman in our first story, you must have an adequate supply of all the building blocks that are necessary for the whole process to proceed as smoothly and efficiently as nature intended. If you've read our earlier books *The Natural Way to Better Babies* and *The Natural Way to a Better Pregnancy* you'll already be aware of the importance of nutrition for every aspect of reproductive health, so you can think of this information as a short refresher course.

If you haven't read those books, the rest of this chapter will serve as a summary.

A BETTER DIET FOR A BETTER BIRTH

A diet of whole, organically grown foods will help to ensure that you have a normal, full-term pregnancy and a healthy baby, so it shouldn't come as too great a surprise to learn that the same sort of diet can also dramatically affect the ease and duration of your labour. Studies of animals show conclusively that those mothers who are deficient in one or more essential nutrients have prolonged labours. But humans are very different from animals, and it's not quite so easy to carry out the same sort of strictly controlled experiments that are conducted on animal populations.

However, careful studies made in the early part of this century by Dr Weston Price, an American dentist, clearly demonstrated that when native communities ate their traditional, unrefined, wholefood diet, they enjoyed general good health. They had good looks, freedom from dental decay, robust immune systems, competent mental function and short labours and easy deliveries.

Once a community changed to eating white flour and products containing sugar, however, there was an overall decline in both physical and mental health and in the efficiency and ease of the birth process.

Other observers noted that medical staff working amongst remote Inuit communities in Northern Canada never saw an Inuit woman give birth—the labour was simply never long enough for the medical attendant to get there in time. The women who had these short, efficient labours were consuming the traditional Inuit diet, and the distinction was made between these women and those who had been exposed to a refined, processed, Western-style diet. The latter had difficult and prolonged labours, which often required transfer to hospital and medical intervention.

Despite the fact that these observations demonstrate a direct link between good nutritional status and an easy birth, little attention is paid to these findings today. Instead of attending to one of the most fundamental factors contributing to protracted labours and difficult births, the medical profession has devised a succession of obstetrical interventions to 'help things along' and 'speed things up'. Unfortunately, in the process of fine-tuning the labour and expediting the birth of a baby, all women, whether experiencing a long and difficult delivery or not, have been caught up in this tinkering process.

But we've already belaboured (pardon the pun) the point about inappropriate obstetrical intervention, so let's go back to the importance of nutrition. An adequate supply of all the nutritional factors, which includes vitamins, trace minerals and essential amino and fatty acids, is needed for your body's and your baby's development during your pregnancy. They're also needed in adequate amounts to ensure the presence of all the complex and interdependent factors required to initiate your labour and continue it efficiently until your baby is born. Adequate nutrition is also essential for both bonding and breast-feeding to proceed smoothly. So let's look now at the specific nutritional factors which can affect labour, birth and bonding. Later in this chapter we'll describe how to modify your diet to obtain optimum levels of these nutrients.

ZINC: FOR A BETTER LABOUR, POSTPARTUM PERIOD AND LACTATION

Zinc is involved in over 200 enzyme systems in the body and has extremely important functions during every aspect of reproduction including labour. It is equally important in the period immediately following the birth, and during the whole period of breast-feeding.

Zinc deficient women have long labours

Zinc is an essential component of collagen and, consequently, of all connective tissue. In women who are zinc deficient, gaps appear in the uterine membrane and this dramatically reduces the efficiency of the uterine contractions. This means that women who are zinc deficient are likely to have long labours due to inefficient contractions.

Zinc battles postnatal depression

Zinc has a number of other functions as well. As your pregnancy nears its end, your body undergoes changes that prepare it for giving birth. Under the influence of hormones, copper levels rise and zinc packs into the placenta. These high copper levels are thought to be one of the factors that trigger the phenomenon of birth, so your body needs an adequate supply of this element. This is usually easily achieved in Australia because drinking water, which has flowed through copper pipes, contains a plentiful supply of this mineral. Zinc deficiency is a much more common problem, and if your zinc levels are low your high copper levels will not return to normal after you've given birth and there's a good chance you'll suffer from postnatal depression. (Zinc and copper are antagonistic minerals—one is needed to balance the other.)

In traditional societies (and in the animal kingdom) zinc deficiency and postnatal depression is rarely a problem because the placenta is usually eaten. This organ is the richest known source of zinc—it contains between 350–600 mg of elemental zinc, depending on its size. When the placenta is eaten, adequate zinc status is very quickly restored, maternal zinc stores are established (very important during breastfeeding), and high copper levels fall back to normal. If you'd like to try this method of re-establishing adequate zinc status, treat the placenta like a piece of liver and fry with garlic, onions and tomatoes. Alternatively, you can try a stew with mushrooms and red wine (go easy on the alcohol though), or blend to make a pâté. (If our recipes don't inspire you, there is an alternative—just keep reading.)

The birth of a baby will certainly bring recognition of one cycle ending, and inevitably, there must be some degree of mourning to accompany that ending. However, the sense of sadness and of leaving something behind should be eclipsed by an incredible sense of fulfilment. This and the anticipation of another, new cycle beginning are what a good birth and appropriate bonding can bring. Nature has designed the whole process in such a way that the birth of a new baby and those early months can, and should be, one of the happiest and most rewarding periods of a woman's life. The birth of a child should bring with it all the joy and exhilaration of falling in love, yet this isn't the case for many women.

Statistics show that up to one third of all birthing women in western society exhibit some degree of postnatal depression. Those statistics tell us that something is seriously amiss. There is no doubt that grieving for a lost birth experience, which can occur if you have a surgically assisted delivery, is a factor. Lack of close family, or other emotional support, and a sense of loss of control, which some women experience after the birth of a child, are other factors which can contribute to this condition. But simply restoring adequate zinc status before the birth of your baby can make a huge difference to whether or not you are affected. Interestingly, the oral contraceptive pill causes high copper and low zinc levels in users, and the rise in pill use corresponds exactly with the rise in the incidence of postnatal depression.

Zinc is important for strong connective tissue

Adequate zinc (as well as plenty of vitamins C and E) will ensure that all connective tissue is strong. Strong connective tissue means that you're protected from pre-term rupture of the membranes and also means that your perineum will stretch readily so you'll be less likely to tear or require an episiotomy. If you have a natural, unmedicated birth, you'll suffer little obvious physical trauma to your body, but don't forget, nutrients are needed for the tissue repair which must take place inside the uterus where the placenta was attached and for the healing of any labial grazes or tears. Betacarotene is another nutrient that can help to prevent pre-term rupture of the membranes.

If you have to undergo an episiotomy, adequate nutritional status is even more vital, since the amount of tissue repair required is significantly increased. If for any reason complications requiring a Caesarean section develop, you will make a much faster recovery, with quicker wound healing and less chance of infection, if you are not suffering from a deficiency of zinc or other essential nutrients. If your baby suffers any injury at birth (e.g. from a forceps delivery) he will also recover more quickly if his nutritional stores are adequate and if he continues to receive plenty of zinc and other nutrients in your breast milk.

Zinc protects against cracked nipples

Adequate zinc levels can also offer protection against cracked nipples. While proper attachment of your newborn to the breast is the surest way to avoid this condition, strong nipple tissue is important too, especially if you have a baby who really likes to suck. The individual temperament of your baby may partly determine the length and pace of your labour as we've already described. This individual temperament can also have a large bearing on your baby's need to nurse at the breast. Some infants are satisfied with brief feeds while others need almost constant oral gratification. If you have one of the latter, their frequent and lengthy nursing at a breast unaccustomed to such things can put a strain on the most robust and zinc-adequate nipple tissue.

Jan and Francesca's sons were all breast-fixated. We remember many lengthy nursing sessions and also remember feeling that we might never be able to detach our children for long enough to leave the house alone again. Fortunately we knew about the importance of adequate zinc status and never suffered from cracked nipples. Despite dire predictions that we would be offering our breasts at the university gates, all the boys eventually weaned themselves (and are now very secure individuals), though Francesca's first son was old enough to be reaching for *Playboy* from the newsagent's stand while calling out 'Tit! Tit!' and Jan's boys were eased into their first days of school with a quick breastfeed.

Adequate zinc for contented babies

If you think that new babies are synonymous with crying, we'd like to assure you that this definitely isn't the case. Achieving and maintaining adequate zinc status before you give birth can ensure that the two don't go hand in hand. The baby who has received adequate zinc in utero and continues to receive adequate zinc after birth is easy to soothe and does not cry excessively.

In contrast, a baby who is zinc deficient is very jittery and may cry inconsolably. Alone, this crying can give a new mother a good reason for being depressed. If the mother is also zinc deficient (which is usually why the baby becomes zinc deficient in the first place) she may be suffering from 'baby blues' or from a more severe case of postnatal depression. This duo—a zinc deficient, depressed mother and a zinc deficient, endlessly crying baby—is caught in a very vicious cycle indeed.

How to ensure adequate zinc status

Perhaps you still can't quite come to grips with the idea of placenta pâté? Relax—there is another option—you can bury the placenta in the garden under a special tree or bush and choose another way to restore zinc status. Zinc supplementation can do the same for your zinc levels as consumption of the placenta. Ideally, a zinc supplement should be taken throughout your pregnancy, but even if you're in the latter stages of that now, you've still got time to do something about restoring your zinc status to adequate levels. First you'll need to undertake the Zinc Taste Test.

The Zinc Taste Test

You'll need a simple solution of zinc sulphate heptahydrate (590mg/100mL) in purified water which you can purchase as a proprietary product from your natural health practitioner, health food store or pharmacy. You need to take 5mL of the solution into your mouth and swish it around for one minute.

If you experience a strong, unpleasant taste promptly, your zinc status is adequate, but you need to maintain those adequate levels. To do this you can supplement with zinc taken in tablet form. Zinc chelate (along with co-factors such as magnesium, manganese, Vitamin B6 and betacarotene) is the most appropriate supplement and this should be taken separately, not with food or any other supplements. (Last thing at night is usually a good time.)

If you experience something more like a dry furry sensation, your zinc status is marginal. If you experience no taste at all then you are zinc deficient, and in both instances you must supplement using the same liquid product you administered for the Taste Test. Alternatively, there are other, more concentrated products that can act quickly to restore zinc status. When you start to experience a strong unpleasant taste promptly, you can revert to supplementing with tablets.

The Taste Test should be carried out at two-monthly intervals during your pregnancy, although if your pregnancy is well advanced, you might benefit from more frequent testing, and from slightly more aggressive supplementation.

THE ZINC TASTE TEST

TEST RESULT	SUPPLEMENT: DOSAGE AND FORM (To be taken separately from food and other supplements)
The taste is strong and prompt (and was also at the previous test)	*One zinc tablet daily of 20–25mg elemental zinc (as amino acid chelate)*
The taste is strong and prompt (as a result of building zinc status since previous test)	*Two zinc tablets daily of 20–25 mg elemental zinc (as amino acid chelate)*
The taste is of medium strength or the response is slightly delayed	*5 mL twice daily*
The taste is slight or the response is delayed	*10 mL twice daily*
There is no taste	*20 mL twice daily*

N.B The liquid measures we give here are only appropriate for the preparation we describe in the text. Other commercial preparations may be more concentrated and an equivalent, smaller dose can be used. Always make sure that your dose of liquid zinc is well diluted with water (250 mL at least). If you need to take higher doses of zinc, re-test at least once a week and adapt the dosage level appropriately.

While it's important that you ensure that your zinc status is adequate, zinc is just one of many essential nutrients which, when present in adequate amounts, can contribute to a better birth and better bonding. Let's have a look at some of the others.

OTHER NUTRIENTS FOR A BETTER BIRTH

Nutrients for your baby's brain development

Unlike most of your baby's organs, which have largely formed by the end of the first trimester, with growth being the main feature of the second and third trimesters, your baby's brain continues to develop throughout the whole pregnancy and for the first three years of life. This development, especially the fine tuning, is dependent on a good supply of the essential fatty acids, omega-3 and omega-6. There is considerable uptake of and demand for these nutrients in the last six weeks of pregnancy, and if a baby misses out on this important phase of development, through premature birth, it is extremely important that the nutrients are delivered to him in the first weeks outside the uterus. The breast milk of a well-nourished mother is rich in these essential fatty acids, but they are usually lacking in infant formulae, although some manufacturers are now aware of the need to ensure their presence. The best supplement to provide you with these nutrients as you approach birth (and during the breastfeeding period) is one which provides a balanced combination of evening primrose oil and deep-sea fish oils. Make sure to buy a reputable brand of this essential fatty acid combination since some fish oils may be contaminated with PCBs (polychlorinated biphenyls), DDT, dioxin and mercury.

Nutrients for practice contractions

Throughout your pregnancy you will experience Braxton-Hicks contractions and in the latter weeks these will increase in frequency and intensity. These contractions are painless—this is simply your uterus having a trial run—but nutrients such as calcium, magnesium and potassium are necessary for these contractions to be really efficient and do some of the work of effacing (thinning) the cervix before true labour starts. In an optimally nourished woman, significant effacement (and dilation) can be achieved before the serious contractions, which really hurt, begin in earnest. As well as an adequate supply of the trace minerals needed for efficient contractions, vitamin E is an important nutrient to ensure that the uterine muscle is strong. Calf muscles are also affected in the pregnancy by a deficiency in calcium and magnesium. If you experience cramping in your legs, you should step up your supplementation.

Nutrients needed to manufacture prostaglandins, hormones and endorphins

The formation of prostaglandins—highly biologically active compounds which trigger hormonal activity vital for labour—is dependent on the presence of an adequate supply of all the essential nutrients. Both you and your baby manufacture prostaglandins and, if you are lacking in key nutrients, your labour will fail to proceed smoothly, because the hormones and chemical transmitters dependent on prostaglandin activity will not be present in sufficient quantities.

To ensure adequate levels of prostaglandins and hormones, keep up your intake of the essential fatty acids, zinc, magnesium, selenium and vitamins B6, C and E. This will ensure that your cervix softens and ripens quickly and that, towards the end of your pregnancy, all your muscles and ligaments relax under the influence of a hormone called relaxin. This complete relaxation allows your pelvis and the birth canal to open fully. (Remember, too, that complete opening is not possible if you're lying flat on your back!)

Your baby will usually assume a head down, anterior lie with his face pointing towards your back-bone. This is the most common position and the most effective for his journey down the birth canal. An inadequate supply of any of the hormones or prostaglandins may cause him to assume a posterior (face pointing towards your tummy), breech (bottom down instead of head down) or transverse (horizontal) lie.

Your body must also manufacture adequate amounts of the hormone oxytocin if your uterus is to contract effectively. Inadequate levels of essential fatty acids and other nutrients, combined with stress (and the resulting production of adrenaline) adversely affect oxytocin production as we've already described in Chapter 2.

During labour, your body manufactures morphine-like substances called endorphins that are natural pain relievers. As we've seen in

Chapter 2, endorphin production can be inhibited by induction and by drugs. Production can also be impaired if your nutritional status is compromised. Magnesium is one of many nutrients necessary to ensure plenty of circulating endorphins that will raise your body's pain threshold.

Nutrients needed for energy

An adequate supply of all the nutritional factors means that you'll have plenty of energy. You'll need it too, because no matter how short and straightforward your labour may be, it's still hard work. Similar to a brisk 6-kilometre hike! But if you're well nourished (and if you're fit and strong), you won't tire readily, and you'll be more likely to participate actively in the birth.

All the B-complex vitamins and minerals such as zinc, magnesium, chromium and manganese are important for energy production because they're involved in the metabolism of complex carbohydrates. The complete metabolic breakdown of these substances ensures a constant supply of glucose. This is the most readily available fuel for all of your body's processes, including muscle contraction.

Nutrients needed for blood clotting

One of the best ways to avoid postpartum haemorrhage is to nurse your baby immediately after birth. Oxytocin, which is the hormone responsible for the let-down reflex during breastfeeding, also causes your uterus to contract and clamp down on itself. But as well as the presence of oxytocin, the essential fatty acids, calcium, manganese and vitamin K are important. Adequate amounts of these nutrients, coupled with early breastfeeding, can ensure appropriate blood clotting and minimal postpartum bleeding.

Nutrients needed after the birth

It's vital to maintain adequate nutritional status after you've given birth to avoid postnatal depression and cracked nipples and to ensure that healing of tears or incisions takes place quickly. And if you have adequate stores of all the essential nutrients, the demands of your new baby won't cause the excessive fatigue that is a characteristic of early (and not so early) postpartum days for many women.

Nutrients needed for maternal instinct

It might come as a surprise to learn that your nutritional status can affect something as fundamental as the instinctive desire to 'mother' which is essential for the survival of the young of any species. Research shows that the essential mineral manganese, through certain enzymes, affects the glandular secretions underlying maternal instinct.

Zinc is another nutrient that is important for ensuring appropriate maternal behaviour. Animal studies have shown that zinc deficient rat mothers will not build nests, will not nurse their young, will not retrieve the young that stray, and may even totally abandon their offspring. While human mothering is a great deal more complex (and extended) than that of animals, the fact that a simple nutritional deficiency can have such a profound effect on instinctive mammalian behaviour is an important observation that again supports the need for adequate nutritional status.

It also leads us to ask some hard questions. The organophosphate pesticides, used routinely in non-sustainable farming operations, block the uptake of manganese from soil, while zinc deficiency is now the most widespread deficiency in the Western world. Could these deficiencies be contributing to a general decline in maternal instinct? Is this decline reflected, in worst instances, in the increasing levels of child abuse and neglect? Is it seen, in less serious cases, as the increasing desire for child care for even the tiniest babies? Is it exhibited, in its most subtle form, as women happy to hand over their birth experience to the medical profession, and their breastfeeding experience to the manufacturers of infant formulae?

We do not for one moment suggest that nutritional factors are the only ones in these equations. But we ask the questions simply to draw your attention to the fact that maternal instinct, along with many other mental and emotional states, is kept balanced and stable, for the most part, by the solid underpinning of sound nutritional status.

Nutrients for nutritious breast milk

The quality of your breast milk depends on your nutritional status too. As already discussed, an adequate supply of zinc in your milk is essential, since babies who are zinc deficient are very difficult to console. The essential fatty acids are also vital. As we've seen, they're important for the development of your baby's brain and also his eyes. Brain development continues at a rapid rate for about three years after birth, so make sure that you eat a really healthy diet and take a supplement which contains the appropriate balance of both omega-3 and omega-6 essential fatty acids while you're breastfeeding.

Since breast milk is undoubtedly the best source of those essential fatty acids (despite the claims of the manufacturers who now add these essential nutrients to artificial formulae), we want to emphasise the importance of breastfeeding for as long as possible. The brain development that continues during your baby's early years highlights the undesirability of early weaning and, indeed, of putting any arbitrary limit on the breastfeeding period at all. Your baby is the best person to judge when he no longer needs breast milk.

We'll talk more of the importance of nutritional status and its relationship to successful breastfeeding and infant growth and development during lactation in our next book *The Natural Way to Better Breastfeeding and Beyond*. Until we've written it, please take our word for it and make sure you're a really well-nourished breastfeeding mother.

We hope this information has convinced you that good nutrition is one of the most important ingredients of a better birth and bonding. Let's look now at what you should be eating (and taking) to ensure your nutritional status is adequate.

Of course, if you've been diligent about your diet throughout your pregnancy and if you've been taking your supplements as our earlier books recommended, then your nutrient levels will already be in the optimum range. But if you've suffered from morning sickness, or if you've been a bit careless about your food intake, you might have depleted your body's nutrient stores. However, it's never too late for a positive approach. Even if you've only got a couple of months or even weeks to go before the big day, you can still do a great deal to improve your intake of all the building blocks your body needs for the labour, birth, bonding and breastfeeding period.

EATING FOR OPTIMAL NUTRITION

Try, wherever possible, to select foods which are fresh, in season, unprocessed and organically grown or fed. Whole, uncontaminated food is high in nutritional value and low in toxins and ideal for you and your baby. To help you make positive choices—and stay away from refined, processed foods which do you no good—you can repeat an affirmation such as *'I am making a positive choice for my health and wellbeing and that of my child'* or *'Better diet, better birth, better baby'*. As a bonus, you'll find that eating well isn't the chore you may have been dreading—organic produce tastes great and these days is widely available. You'll find some helpful sources at the end of this book.

The Zone Diet

Just as important as what you should be eating (and what you should be avoiding) is the appropriate balance of all those good foods. When you achieve the appropriate ratio of carbohydrate, protein and fat, you balance two key hormones—insulin and glucagon. When you do this, nutritionists say you're *in the zone*. Try to stay *in the zone* for a better birth, bonding and breastfeeding experience.

You can start by thinking of insulin as the saving hormone—it tells your body to save fat. Glucagon, on the other hand, is the spending hormone—it takes energy from the fat cells to be used as fuel. When these two hormones are well balanced, your blood sugar levels won't fluctuate. Stable blood sugar levels mean you will be less likely to suffer from fatigue and emotional instability. They will ensure that you have plenty of energy and increased endurance for your labour, and promote a quick recovery and faster healing of any wounds. They also mean your baby will receive a constant supply of glucose for his energy needs.

Let's look at the steps involved in achieving that desirable ratio.

First, work out your daily protein requirements. At each meal you need an amount of protein that can fit on the palm of your hand (and be no thicker than the palm of your hand). Now increase that amount by ⅓ (for your pregnancy), by a further ¼ for light physical activity, by ⅓ for moderate activity (30 minutes of exercise three days per week) and by ½ for strenuous activity (60 minutes of exercise five days per week). You can use either primary (animal) or secondary (plant) protein.

Primary protein is complete protein; it contains all the essential amino acids. The main primary proteins include fish, chicken, eggs, dairy foods and red meat. Let's look at which are best for a pregnant woman.

- **Fish** You should eat fish at least 2–3 times weekly. Fish is low in saturated fats and high in essential fatty acids. Especially beneficial are the deep-sea, ocean and cold-water fish, which are also less polluted, e.g. mackerel, mullet, salmon, taylor, trevally and sardines. You should avoid large fish, which may contain high levels of mercury, e.g. tuna, shark and swordfish. Fresh fish is definitely preferable to tinned or frozen fish.

- **Chicken** Eat free-range and organically-fed poultry only. Note that the two are not necessarily the same thing, as some free-range poultry are fed hormones and antibiotics. Trim the skin to avoid unhealthy fats.

- **Eggs** Most expectant mothers should eat a maximum of 2–3 eggs per week. However, if you are confident you are not allergic or sensitive to eggs, and they don't cause gastro-intestinal or digestive problems, such as gas or constipation, you can increase your consumption as eggs are a good protein source. Make sure they are from free-range and organically-fed poultry.

- **Dairy foods** Avoid cow's milk and cheese. Cow's milk products can create mucus and congestion in your gut (which can compromise your absorption of nutrients). Natural acidophilus, non-flavoured yoghurt is a good choice, as are goat's or soya milk and cheese.

- **Red meat** Eat red meat in moderation. Lean meat (with the fat trimmed) and game meat are best. Unless you are certain that the animal has been organically fed, avoid organ meats, sausage and mince (which are often made from the organs). Organ meats contain high levels of pesticides and hormones as they are the detoxifying routes for the animal. Some butchers make their own gourmet sausages (which contain more meat, although they are still high in fat), and if you want mince you can get the butcher to mince a selected lean cut on site. You should avoid delicatessen meats, which are high in fats, offal content and toxic preservatives.

Secondary proteins are incomplete proteins as they do not contain the full range of essential amino acids, but by combining two of the food groups listed below during each day, you will have a complete protein source, as each group contains a different range of amino acids.

- **Nuts** These should be raw, unsalted and fresh. Store nuts in the refrigerator, away from light, and eat them within two weeks of purchase. (Nuts should never taste bitter as this means the oil they contain has gone rancid.) Alternatively, you can buy unshelled nuts and remove the shell as needed. Nuts are a good source of beneficial oils and many nutrients, and you can use them in stir-fries, salads, pasta dishes, and as a snack.

- **Grains and seeds** Whole grains are a source of plant protein as well as a source of carbohydrate. Eat whole grains such as wholemeal bread, wholemeal pasta (green-coloured pasta might be refined white pasta with dye added) and organically grown grains whenever possible. In the case of rice, Basmati (which is white rice), actually has a lower glycaemic index than brown rice, although it's not as nutritious. (We'll talk more about glycaemic index in just a moment.) You should avoid refined flour products such as cakes, biscuits and pastries because they leach nutrients from your body's stores. Always read bread packets carefully and avoid those which contain preservatives or other additives.

- **Legumes and pulses** Lentils, dried beans, soya, tofu and tempeh are also sources of vegetable protein and have the added benefit of acting as detoxifiers. However, you should avoid those brands of soy products that might contain genetically engineered beans or high levels of aluminium. Try to get the soy products that clearly state 'Contains no genetically modified soybeans'. It pays to check labels carefully.

Once you've selected your protein portion, the next step is to add your carbohydrates. There are two types of carbohydrates—risk-reducing (low glycaemic) and risk-promoting (high glycaemic) carbohydrates. The category into which a particular food falls depends on the amount of carbohydrate present in the food and the amount of fibre it contains. Low carbohydrate and high fibre/water content foods are risk-reducing and it is those foods you should select whenever possible.

Low-risk vegetables and pulses include asparagus, avocado, bok choy, broccoli, brussels sprouts, cabbage, capsicum, cauliflower, chick-peas, cucumber, eggplant, kidney beans, lentils, lettuce, mushrooms, onion, spinach and tomatoes. You should eat lots of vegetables from this category every day. Select a wide variety, especially those that are dark green and leafy or red and orange, as well as avocado (which is also a good source of essential fatty acids). Eat both raw and cooked vegetables on a regular basis. You can steam, stir-fry or dry-bake them, but do not cook or defrost with microwaves, as these destroy protein structures and the enzymes that are required for the proper assimilation of vitamins and minerals.

There are lots of interesting green leafy vegetables to choose from for your salads, although remember that pale lettuce is not highly nutritious. All vegetables except potatoes can be eaten raw, so try tossing raw mushrooms, cabbage and cauliflower into your salad bowl. Add chopped fresh herbs like parsley and watercress for interest and flavour, and because they are high in minerals. Seaweed (organic only) is a highly nutritious vegetable which can be added to soups, stir-fries, etc.

You might like to try vegetable juices as a great way of ensuring adequate vegetable intake. Carrot, celery and beetroot are a popular combination, but any vegetable you have in your fridge can be added.

Low-risk fruits include apples, apricots, berries, grapes, melons, oranges, peaches, pineapple, strawberries, cherries and pears. You should eat no more than 2–3 pieces of fruit daily (because of the high fruit sugar content). This includes fruit that is juiced, which should be diluted half and half with purified water. Avoid dried fruit which is high in sugar and usually contains preservatives.

The moderate-risk foods which can still be eaten, but in smaller amounts, include baked beans, corn, carrots, peas, potatoes, squash, sweet potato, bananas, dates, figs, mango, papaya, fruit juices, pastas, breads, cereal grains and condiments (such as tomato sauce and chutney).

Once you've selected your protein and carbohydrates you need to add healthy fats. Fats or oils are a vital component of each meal, since every wall of every cell in your body contains a lipid (fat) layer. Fats are also necessary to tell your brain that you have had enough to eat. They also reduce your blood sugar and insulin response to a meal and are a very important part of achieving the balance between insulin and glucagon. Here are some healthy fats and oils and suggestions for using them.

- For dressings and sauces try olive, flax, pumpkin, walnut, canola, safflower and sunflower oils (all cold pressed). These are high in fatty acids if they aren't heated. They should be kept out of the light (in dark containers) and in the fridge (except olive oil). You can add lemon, pepper, garlic and herbs to dressings.

- For cooking try olive, sesame and canola oils which do not saturate on heating.

- Use flax, pumpkin, sesame and sunflower seeds in salads and cooking, or for snacks.

- Walnuts, hazelnuts and almonds are also good in salads or as snacks.

- Avocado can be used in salads or mashed as a dip or spread.

- Try soya mayonnaise with your salads or sandwiches.

You can have snacks between meals as you shouldn't go more than four hours without food. Just work out the appropriate proportions of protein, carbohydrate and fat as outlined above, but halve your protein allowance at snack time.

Finally, you need to drink plenty of purified water—between 8–12 glasses (2–3 litres)—every day. Spring (still) water is a reasonable substitute. Mineral (sparkling) water is acceptable occasionally, but may be high in salt. Unpurified tap water is high in toxins and heavy metals that are concentrated, not destroyed, by boiling. Make sure that you drink in between meals so that the water doesn't interfere with your digestion, and if you're already up and down several times during the night to empty your bladder, limit your increased water intake to the early part of the day.

What to avoid

- Avoid saturated fats, including butter and margarine, heated and animal fats, which compete with EFAs and are a reservoir for toxins and pollutants (which are fat-soluble). These will upset your prostaglandin/hormone/mineral balance. Margarine is worse than butter—it saturates during processing and is full of chemicals. Try avocado, banana, hummus, or nut spreads, but only if they are fresh and refrigerated and kept away from light.

- Avoid eating fried food, except stir-fries. Cook with olive oil, which is a mono-unsaturated oil that will not saturate on heating. Canola and sesame oils are acceptable alternatives.

- Avoid sugar and all sweet things, including honey, sugar substitutes, undiluted fruit juices, cakes, biscuits, pastries and soft drinks. Sugar leaches essential nutrients from your body, and increases your insulin response. Read labels carefully. Sugar has lots of other names, for example, dextrose, glucose, fructose (and other words ending in '-ose'), corn starch, malt, maple syrup, molasses, etc.

- Only add salt 'to taste'. Do not use it routinely in cooking or on food. Use rock, sea or Celtic salt rather than ordinary table salt. Avoid highly salted, pre-prepared foods.

- Avoid junk foods—they usually fall into high saturated fat, high salt, high sugar, low nutrient categories. Read labels carefully and avoid additives.

- Avoid alcohol completely—it is toxic to the foetus and leaches nutrients from your body.

- Avoid coffee—it is related to problems in pregnancy, including miscarriage, and it compromises foetal development. We don't recommend decaffeinated coffee because of the chemicals used to remove the caffeine. Even if decaffeinated through a natural, water-based process, the coffee will contain other harmful constituents which become more active during this procedure. Cereal-based substitutes and dandelion root coffee are acceptable, but check that they do not contain added sugar. Or you can drink a maximum of 2 cups of weak, naturally low caffeine (not decaffeinated) tea daily. Green and herb teas are preferable.

SUPPLEMENTATION FOR OPTIMAL NUTRITION

You might think that nutritional supplements are superfluous if you have a healthy diet and are staying *in the zone* as we've recommended. It can be very difficult, however, to obtain all the nutrients you need for a better birth and bonding from your diet alone because of various environmental and lifestyle factors. For instance, even if you eat only organic whole foods now, you'll still have nutrient deficits to make up from years of eating non-organic produce grown or grazed on depleted soils and dipped or drenched in a variety of chemicals. It's inevitable too that you'll be exposed to pollution, and your body will require extra essential nutrients to detoxify the heavy metals, chemicals and additives found in many foods, the water supply and the air. Stress, allergies and illness also significantly increase your requirements of essential nutrients. And of course every individual is biochemically different and it may simply be impossible for some of you to receive an adequate nutrient intake from diet alone (no matter how nutritious it is).

So we strongly recommend you take the following daily dosages of supplements.

SUPPLEMENT	DAILY DOSAGE
Vitamin A	10 000 IU, or 6 mg betacarotene. Choose mixed carotenoids if available. This dose of vitamin A has been shown to be completely safe in pregnancy, but should not be exceeded.

SUPPLEMENT	DAILY DOSAGE
Vitamin B complex	B1, B2, B3, B5, B6: 50 mg each B12: 400 mcg Biotin: 200 mcg Choline, inositol, PABA: 25 mg Folic acid: 500 mcg (0.5 mg). Increase this to 1000 mcg (1 mg) daily if you have had a previous miscarriage, if there is a history of neural tube defects in your family, or if you are over 40 years of age
Vitamin C	1000–2000 mg (1–2 g). Take the higher dose temporarily if you are suffering from infection
Bioflavonoids	500–1000 mg (helpful for preventing miscarriage and excessive bleeding)
Vitamin D	200 IU
vitamin E	500 IU (increasing to 800 IU during last trimester)
Calcium	800 mg (increasing to 1200 mg if symptoms such as leg cramps indicate an increased need)
Magnesium	400 mg daily (half the dose of calcium)
Potassium	15 mg or as cell salt (potassium chloride, 3 tablets)
Iron	Supplement only if need is proven; dosage depends on serum ferritin levels (stored iron) and supplement should be chelated and organic. If levels < 30 mcg per litre, take 30 mg If levels < 45 mcg per litre, take 20 mg If levels < 60 mcg per litre, take 10 mg
Manganese	10 mg
Zinc	20–60 mg. Take it on an empty stomach, and separately from other supplements. The dosage level depends on the result of Zinc Taste Test. See earlier in this chapter

SUPPLEMENT	DAILY DOSAGE
Chromium	100–200 mcg daily (upper limit for those with sugar cravings, and in last trimester, when gestational diabetes can become a problem, especially if not supplemented throughout pregnancy)
Selenium	100–200 mcg (upper limit for those exposed to high levels of heavy metal or chemical pollution). Seleno-methionine is the most stable and useful form of this mineral. Sodium selenite is less useful and must be taken separately from vitamin C and zinc. You may need a prescription for the higher doses in Australia
Iodine	75 mcg (or eat organic seaweed or take 150 mg of kelp instead)
Acidophilus/Bifidus	Half to one teaspoonful of each, one to three times daily (upper limits for those who suffer from thrush)
Evening primrose oil/ flaxseed oil	500 mg two to three times daily
EPA/DHA (deep sea fish oils)	500 mg two to three times daily (especially if your diet contains little deep-sea fish)
Garlic	2000–5000 mg (higher levels for those exposed to toxins)
Silica	20 mg
Copper	1–2 mg (but only if zinc levels are adequate)
Hydrochloric acid and digestive enzymes	For those with digestive problems. There are numerous proprietary preparations that contain an appropriate combination of active ingredients. Ask your health practitioner for guidance and take as directed
Co-enzyme Q10	10 mg

Ideally, supplementation should begin before conception and continue throughout your pregnancy, but if you have only a short time to go before your big day and have not yet taken any supplements, don't despair. Do start now, but note that you may need to add some nutrients in slighter greater quantities. Since calcium and magnesium are required for uterine (and all muscle) contractions, a crash course in these two minerals may be helpful. You can double the dosages we give here at no risk. The celloids, or tissue salts, calcium phosphate and magnesium phosphate are absorbed very quickly, and may be useful as labour approaches.

Remember to check your zinc and stored iron (ferritin) levels regularly throughout pregnancy and as you approach labour, as these two very important minerals compete with each other, so it's necessary to be quite clear about their status so you can supplement accordingly. The Zinc Taste Test and a blood test for serum ferritin levels will indicate whether the levels of these minerals are in the appropriate range.

If you are somewhat alarmed or overwhelmed by the length and seeming complexity of our list of recommended supplements, rest assured there are a number of multivitamin and mineral formulae available which contain a combination of nutrients. You won't have to take and store hundreds of tablets and potions, just a few. Your natural health practitioner is the best person to help you or, if this is not possible, your local health food shop or pharmacy. (If you are interested in finding out more about supplements or have specific questions, you'll find a lot more information in our previous books *The Natural Way to Better Babies* and *The Natural Way to a Better Pregnancy*.)

Remember to take your supplements daily for, as we hope we've made clear, all nutrients have an important role to play during labour, birth and beyond.

Exercise for a better birth

We've explained the importance of adequate nutritional status in achieving a better birth, and how traditional diets, which were of whole, unrefined foods, grown on healthy soil, helped to ensure an easy labour and delivery. Hand in hand with those traditional diets went traditional lifestyles, radically different from today's, which also affected how easily women gave birth.

Women from traditional or tribal communities led very active lives. Their days were usually a succession of quite demanding physical tasks. They worked in the fields sowing seed, they weeded the furrows and harvested the crops. They winnowed the grain, then ground it by hand. They chopped, kneaded and pounded various other foodstuffs. They fetched water from the stream or the well and washed all bedding and clothing by hand. They gathered and plaited thatch for their roofs or made mud bricks for their homes.

If they were from nomadic or itinerant tribes they gathered nuts, seeds, fruit, roots and tubers and collected wood and animal dung to fuel their fires. They might walk many kilometres, frequently with a load tied to their backs or balanced on their heads.

Whether the women came from settled or nomadic tribes, whether they lived in villages or yurts, they spun, wove, cooked and cleaned. During their child-bearing years these women invariably worked at their myriad daily tasks with a baby attached to their body in some sort of sling or papoose. They never considered putting their baby down. If they needed a rest from carrying him they would simply hand him to another family member for a while.

These women had no corner store, motor car, running water, vacuum cleaner, washing machine or dishwasher. They had no pram, stroller, carry-cot or bouncinette, so their level of physical activity was vastly different from ours today. Their muscles were strong and also very flexible, they were used to hard and sustained physical work and this was reflected in how they laboured and gave birth to their babies.

BENEFITS OF REGULAR EXERCISE DURING PREGNANCY

While it's impossible to revert to such a lifestyle, it's certainly desirable during your pregnancy to initiate or maintain a level of physical activity that will strengthen all muscle groups and improve your cardiovascular fitness. The advantages for you and your baby of regular aerobic exercise include better delivery of oxygen and nutrients to the placenta and foetus, more efficient circulation, lower blood pressure, less likelihood of varicose veins, haemorrhoids and constipation and improved stamina and endurance. Since the amount of muscle mass in your body determines your basal metabolic rate, regular muscle strengthening exercise can help to ensure that your weight gain is not excessive. It will also mean more calcium is retained in your bones. This means reduced risk of osteoporosis later in life.

BENEFITS OF REGULAR EXERCISE DURING LABOUR

If you exercise regularly you'll enjoy benefits during your labour as well. Labour is aptly named—it's hard physical work. Just as you feel better during a run, a brisk walk, or other training session if your body is accustomed to regular activity, the same will apply to your labour. Not only will your body be better able to withstand the physical demands that labour places upon it, your labour will be shorter and easier if you've exercised regularly throughout your pregnancy. As well as the usual aerobic and muscle strengthening activities, a third form of exercise which is more labour specific—practising positions and movements for an active birth—if undertaken regularly throughout your pregnancy, will contribute significantly towards a better labour by easing pain and assisting your baby's passage down the birth canal.

BEFORE YOU GET STARTED

We will look at these three forms of exercise more closely in just a moment, but first, there are a few things you should always remember whenever you begin your exercise program.

- Warm up.

- Take it easy at first.

- Slow down if necessary.

- Stay cool—keep well hydrated (drink plenty of purified water).

- Choose an exercise which is comfortable, calming (and cushioning if you're in the latter stages of pregnancy).

- Accommodate your changing size and shape.

- Avoid rapid changes in direction and bouncing during exercise.

- Avoid lying on your belly.

- After four months gestation avoid prolonged exercise while lying on your back.

- Always try to maintain correct posture.

- Don't hold your breath; breathe continuously while exercising.

- Cool down, stretch out.

- Never over-stretch; control the movement.

- Never exercise through any pain or discomfort.

🏃 Consult your doctor if you experience any unusual symptoms such as persistent contractions, vaginal discharge, sudden swelling, headache, palpitations, dizziness or marked fatigue.

AEROBIC EXERCISE

An aerobic exercise routine should consist of three or four sessions every week in which you work to improve your cardiovascular (heart–lung) fitness. Each session should be of at least 30 minutes duration, but you should work at a maximum heart rate of 140–150 beats per minute for no more than 15 consecutive minutes during each session.

If you start your aerobic exercise routine early in your pregnancy, the chances of maintaining it right up to the time of the birth are very good. If you're just reading our advice and nearing the end of your pregnancy, it's never too late to get started, but we suggest that you limit your exercise to power walking or swimming, preferably in a sea-water pool which contains lower levels of chemicals. Walking stimulates Braxton-Hicks contractions. These lead to the production of the hormone relaxin that loosens your ligaments in preparation for giving birth. Some midwives report that those women who experience lots of Braxton-Hicks contractions during their pregnancy have a much shorter labour. The kicking action of freestyle swimming works the pelvic area and is preferable to breaststroke.

MUSCLE STRENGTHENING EXERCISES

Major muscle groups

Muscle strengthening exercises should be done with at least the same frequency as your aerobic exercise. More lean muscle means less body fat, smaller fluctuations in blood sugar levels and reduced likelihood of bone loss during your pregnancy. Strengthening your back, buttock and abdominal muscles is particularly important since these form a supportive girdle around your lower body. If these muscles are strong, your advancing pregnancy is less likely to cause backache, and these same strong muscles mean you'll tire much less readily when you're carrying your newborn in some sort of sling. As we've already pointed out, a strong, fit body will labour more efficiently and this is what you're particularly interested in for the moment.

If you attend a fitness centre, you can ask a qualified instructor to show you specific resistant exercises that are suitable during pregnancy. These can be done using either free weights or the fixed weight machines. If weight training conjures up visions of steroid popping, sweating, muscle bound meat-heads pumping iron you might prefer to do your muscle building in privacy. If this is the case, Jan's business partner at Balmain Wellness Centre has the answer for you. The *TUBE-TRAIN* exercise system is easy to use and works every muscle group. It's also completely portable and comes complete with instructional brochure and workout video (see Contacts and Resources). Alternatively, you can purchase a small set of hand weights, or you can substitute two bottles filled with water and use these as weights. Below are some examples of muscle strengthening exercises. Repeat each exercise 10 times, then have a rest for 60 seconds. This is called one set. Repeat the sequence. As you become stronger you can increase the number of repetitions and the number of sets you perform at each session.

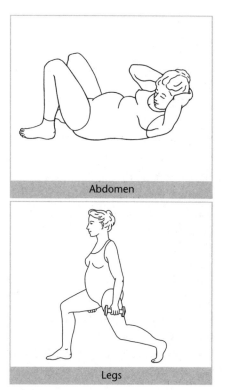

Abdomen

Lie on your back, feet flat on the floor close to your buttocks. Support your head with your hands, making sure you don't pull up on your neck. Lift your head and shoulders and twist to the left. Return to the starting position and repeat, twisting to the right.

Abdomen

Legs

Start with feet shoulder-width apart. Take a good step back on to the ball of that foot. Looking straight ahead, bend your front knee and drop your hips until your thigh is parallel to the floor. Return to the starting position by pushing up with your front leg. Repeat for the other leg.

Legs

Arms

Stand with your feet slightly apart and elbows locked into your sides. Curl the weights towards your shoulder, contracting your biceps. Release slowly, keeping your elbows fixed by your side as you go. If you prefer, you can alternate arms.

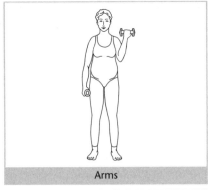
Arms

Chest

Stand with your feet shoulder-width apart. Keeping your elbows high, push the weights away from your body. Return slowly to the starting position.

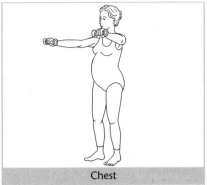
Chest

Shoulders

Stand with feet apart (you may be more comfortable with one foot slightly in front of the other). Lift your elbows sideways to shoulder-height, keeping your arms bent. At the finish position your hands should be slightly lower than your elbows and tilted so that your little fingers are slightly higher than your thumbs.

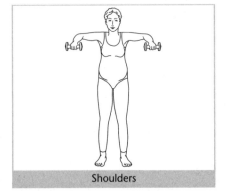
Shoulders

Pelvic floor exercises

Another very important type of muscle strengthening exercise is Kegel, or pelvic floor, exercise. Unlike your biceps, triceps, calves and quadriceps, these muscles are invisible and perhaps that explains why they're often forgotten. They form a sort of diaphragm, separating your pelvic cavity from the perineal area. They have a sphincter-like action on the urethra, the rectum and the birth canal, which all pass through them. Consequently your pelvic floor muscles are involved when you empty your bladder and your bowels and also when you give birth.

If these muscles are weak, they can be stretched and weakened further when your baby passes through them to be born. Weakened pelvic floor muscles mean that you will pee involuntarily every time you laugh, sneeze, cough, jump or run! Apart from the fact that strong pelvic floor muscles have a positive role to play in the birthing process (see below), they also mean that you won't suffer from incontinence, which is very distressing and debilitating.

To perform Kegel exercises, you don't require a personal trainer, there's no need to make a trip to the gym or the swimming pool, you don't even have to change your clothing. But you must remember to do them. We suggest you make several big cut-outs of the letter 'K' and stick them up around the house. Whenever you see these letters, they'll act as a reminder. Janette is so conditioned to this response (she's a bit like Pavlov's dog) that she's instantly doing her Kegels as she types this 'K'. Here's what you do.

First of all you need to visualise these important muscles. They are a sling-like band which forms the base of your vagina, anus and urethra. To identify the feeling of exercising them, next time you want to pee just try to stop the flow of urine in mid-stream. Got it? Then relax the muscles and you've just done your first pelvic floor exercise. Easy isn't it? (Of course we don't want you to continue to do the exercises when you pee, that's just until you get the feel of what to do.) But because Kegels are so easy, they're also easy to forget. That's when those 'K's scattered around the house can be an invaluable and insistent prompt.

It's also important that you try to increase the number of contractions that you perform each time—start with five and work up. You should also increase the length of time for which you hold the contraction—aim for at least five seconds each. Do them whenever you see that 'K' and do them even when you don't. When you're sitting in the car or on the train or bus is a good time. Count how many repetitions you can do while you're watching telly.

There's also another version of this exercise. Think of your pelvic floor muscles as a lift. Take the lift up several floors, making sure that you stop at each floor. You can call out the stops as you go: 'Lingerie, maternity wear, nursery furniture, children's toys, slim-line fashions, back to school!' Then take the lift down, stopping again at each floor.

Finally, when you reach the ground floor, continue to the basement. To do this you must release your pelvic floor muscles completely. This is what you do when you urinate or empty your bowels, and it's exactly how you'll use those muscles in the second stage of labour.

As Kegel exercises tone and strengthen your perineum, they will also protect against tearing and the need for an episiotomy. To avoid perineal damage it's also important to practice squatting and to resist the urge to push too hard as your baby's head is crowning. You may also find it helpful to massage your perineum in the weeks leading up to the birth or during labour. For best effect, follow these steps:

- Wash your hands and sit or lean back in a comfortable position.

- If your vagina is dry, use a natural lubricant, such as olive oil or a natural massage oil.

- Place your thumbs about 3–4 cm inside your vagina. Press downwards and to the sides at the same time. Gently and firmly keep stretching until you feel a slight burning, tingling or stinging sensation.

- Hold the pressure steady until the area becomes a little numb, and the tingling subsides (about two minutes).

- For the next three to four minutes, massage slowly and gently, all around the lower half of your vagina and perineum (avoiding the urinary opening to prevent infection).

- As you massage, keep pulling gently outwards, with your thumbs locked inside the lower part of your vagina, stretching the tissue and skin in preparation for birth.

Incorporating essential oils will make the massage particularly effective. *Lavender* is most effective and can be applied in an oil base or combined with vitamin E cream, which is itself very helpful. *St John's Wort* is a herb which can be made into an oil (not an essential oil), by covering the leaves and flowers of the fresh plant with vegetable oil (such as olive) and exposing to the sun for six weeks. Make sure the oil completely covers the plant to stop it growing mould. You can often find this oil for sale in health food shops, where it is sometimes called *Hypericum* oil, which is the botanical name for the herb. Other useful herbs to apply as an ointment, cream or oil (to keep the perineum healthy and elastic) are *Calendula* and *Comfrey*.

The homoeopathic remedy *Arnica* will also help to prepare your perineum, and prevent bruising. (See Chapter 7 for more on how to use this remedy.)

EXERCISES FOR AN ACTIVE BIRTH

The third type of exercises that you should be doing in preparation for your labour are those which will help you to have an active birth (as opposed to the passive experience you will have if you are confined to bed in a semi-recumbent, or worse still, lithotomy (feet up in stir-rups) position).

As we've shown in Chapter 2, there are huge benefits for both you and your baby if you stay active and upright while you're in labour. If you are free to move around you will intuitively assume the best posi-tion to help ease the pain and assist your baby's journey down the birth canal. Giving birth is completely instinctive when you are able to choose how and where you labour. Those instinctive movements (and sounds) are not only powerful, but they leave you in no doubt about your body's ability to do the job for which it was designed.

If you've been stretching throughout your pregnancy, or if you've been practising yoga, you should be very flexible. Otherwise you'll probably find that, due to an increasingly inactive lifestyle, your body's full range of movement is restricted and your flexibility is reduced, so you won't assume some of the most useful positions easily. If you want to recover your full flexibility and feel absolutely comfortable in the various birthing positions, you'll need to practise them well in advance of going into labour. We'll look first at the various positions you may want to use during labour, and how to practise them, then at some more general forms of exercise which are also a terrific preparation for active birth.

Squatting
Squatting confers lots of benefits. It can lengthen and tone your back, buttock and pelvic floor muscles, it can prevent constipation, can correctly position your uterus and growing baby and regular squatting

will encourage your baby's head to become engaged in the pelvic inlet in the last weeks of your pregnancy.

Squatting is the position in which nature designed you to give birth. When you squat, the birth canal is fully open, the tissues of your perineum are most relaxed, the blood flow to the whole area (and to your baby) is improved and it allows you to feel really open, and physically, as well as mentally, ready to give birth.

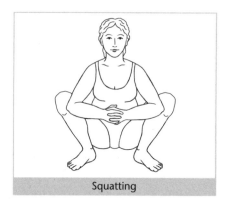

Squatting

You might find this position quite uncomfortable at first. Thanks to high heels and sit down toilets, your ankle joints and Achilles tendons may be very stiff, and squatting with your feet flat on the floor in a position that native women assume so readily and for such extended periods is a position you'll have to work hard to re-learn. You'll probably feel more comfortable in a supported squat to begin with. Try holding onto a friend or a piece of furniture (see diagram 1), or squatting on a pile of books or telephone directories (see diagram 2).

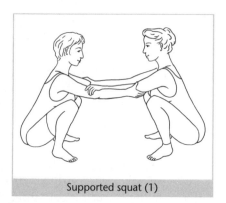

Supported squat (1)

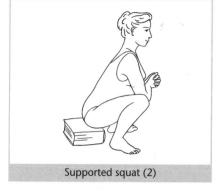

Supported squat (2)

Standing

You might wonder why we suggest you practise standing, but standing during labour is a bit different—it usually becomes a sort of rocking and swaying movement. Practise this with your feet planted firmly, about shoulder width apart, and experience how good it feels to rotate your hips like a belly dancer. Rotate them in one direction, then reverse the movement.

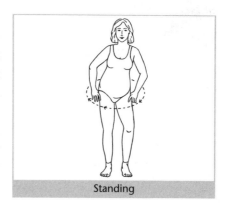

Standing

Supported standing

Leaning forward against a wall or hanging around a support person's neck can be a comfortable position during labour. The wall can support your weight indefinitely of course, but your partner will need some practice to give you support in this position. He must bend his knees and drop his shoulders while you clasp your hands around his neck, hang down and allow your body to relax completely.

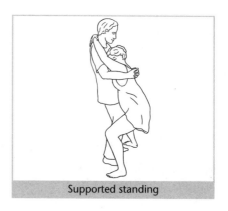

Supported standing

Kneeling

Kneel with your knees about 30 cm apart and your back straight. You might want to put a folded towel or blanket under your knees if the floor is hard. With your hands on your hips, rotate your pelvis as you did in the standing position. Reverse the direction of the rotation.

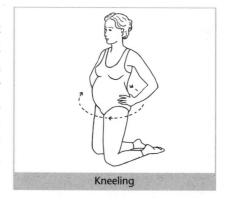

Kneeling

Half kneeling

Bring one knee off the blanket and step forward with that leg so that it now makes a right angle with the floor. You can rock backwards and forwards in this position and change legs as well. This position is particularly helpful for encouraging dilation of your cervix.

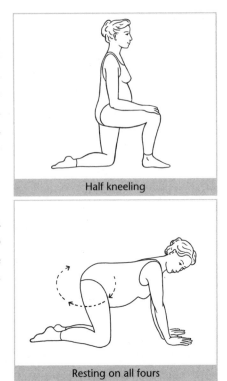

Half kneeling

On all fours

From the kneeling position (above) you can readily move into the all fours position. The same rotation of your pelvis can be practised in both directions.

Resting on all fours

You can further vary this position by exhaling as you arch your back upward while keeping your head down. You should hold this position briefly, breathing naturally. Then, lifting your head up, inhale as you arch downward, curving your lower back. This exercise strengthens your uterus and eases lower back strain.

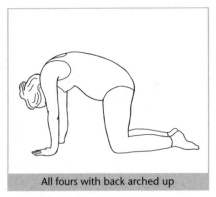

All fours with back arched up

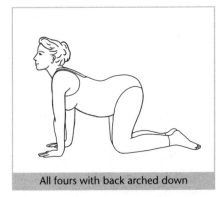

All fours with back arched down

During labour, getting down on all fours like this can help if your baby has assumed a posterior lie or if your contractions become very intense. You can easily deliver your baby while positioned this way. Sometimes you might find it more comfortable to lean forward into a low bed or a pile of pillows, and while on all fours you can also rock back and forth onto your calves if your belly comfortably allows it (see The Child's Pose diagram).

Stretching and yoga to facilitate an active birth

In our last book *The Natural Way to a Better Pregnancy* we described some yoga poses that can help to prepare your body for giving birth. We'd like to repeat them here because they're all so beneficial. They can be used throughout the entire pregnancy and regular practice will facilitate an active birth and ensure an easier delivery. Even if your pregnancy is well advanced, you can still benefit from practising every day.

Baddha Konasana (Supta): The cobbler pose

Sit on the floor with the soles of your feet together, heels as close as possible to your perineum (that's the area between your anus and vulva), with a folded blanket under your feet. Press your toes open against a wall. Then lie back, with a folded blanket supporting your head and neck if you wish. Initially, you should try to hold this pose for 2 minutes, building to 5, 10, then 15 minutes. This posture is great for creating internal space within the pelvic cavity which can facilitate labour and birth. When you're ready to get up, use your left hand to manually lift the left knee over to the right knee and allow your body to roll to the right, finally coming up on your hands and knees.

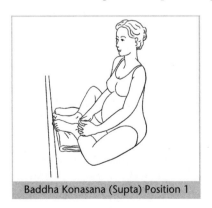
Baddha Konasana (Supta) Position 1

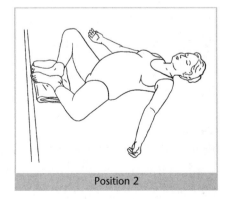
Position 2

Virabhadrasana II: The second warrior pose

This is a standing posture and very useful for increasing strength that will be helpful when you're giving birth. Stand with your back against a wall for support. Place your feet about a metre apart, pointing your right foot away from you and with the left turned in slightly. With your right knee in line with the second toe of your right foot, slowly bend the right knee until it forms a right angle. Hold your arms out straight against the wall at shoulder height, and keep the back leg strong with the knee pulled up. Build to 30 seconds. Come up slowly, keeping the right knee in line with the second right toe on the way up to avoid knee strain. Repeat on the other side.

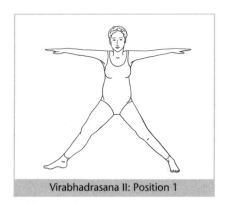
Virabhadrasana II: Position 1

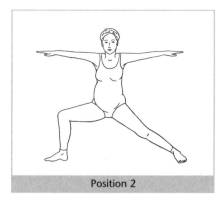
Position 2

Upavista Konasana

Position a chair in front of you, then sit on the floor, with straight legs open comfortably (but not as wide as they will go). Press your heels away, push into your feet, keep your toes turned up. Use the chair to lift your body up. Aim to get your thigh bones closer to the floor. Build up to 3 minutes.

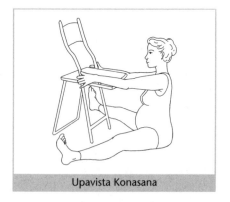
Upavista Konasana

Virasana (Supta)

Kneel with your feet apart, sitting between your feet with a folded blanket under your buttocks. Make sure your feet are facing straight back. When this posture becomes comfortable, lean back, either against a chair, or on folded blankets, bolsters or supportive cushions. Build gradually to 10 minutes. Come up slowly.

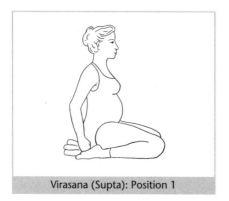

Virasana (Supta): Position 1

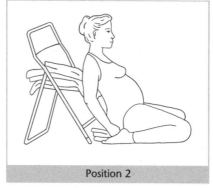

Position 2

If you've been stretching and practising these poses already, you might like to vary your routine now by including some additional postures.

Backward bending

Stand with your feet about shoulder-width apart and place your hands on your hips. Bend back slowly, adjusting for your changing centre of gravity as you go. Relax your head and shoulders then return slowly to the starting position.

Forward bending

From backward bending you can gently move into forward bending. Keep your knees slightly bent, spread your legs apart to accommodate your belly, relax your head and shoulders and just hang down.

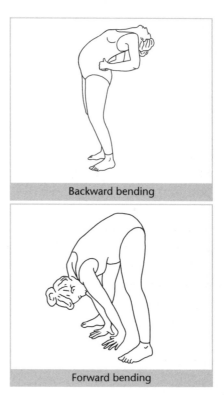

Backward bending

Forward bending

Half headstand

Headstands and shoulderstands are very helpful during pregnancy, as they rest your back and lower abdominals and the muscles in your legs. However, we don't recommend that you attempt these poses for the first time now. Even if you're experienced in performing these asanas, you may still prefer to perform the half-headstand, using a wall for support.

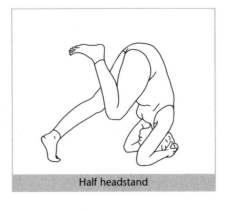

Half headstand

Modified shoulderstand

This is a great way to take the weight off your legs. Lying with your buttocks against the wall, and using your hands for support, stretch your legs up until they are straight. Then practise taking one leg at a time off the wall.

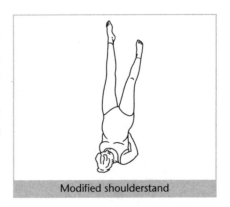

Modified shoulderstand

Forward bend (from the sitting position)

Sit with your legs apart. Bend forward from the hips, spreading your thighs to accommodate your belly. You may be able to hold onto your toes as your flexibility increases.

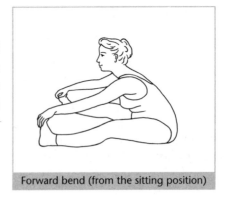

Forward bend (from the sitting position)

Crescent moon

Kneel on the floor, then step forward with one leg. Placing your hands on your forward knee for extra support, bend back slowly and carefully. Relax your head.

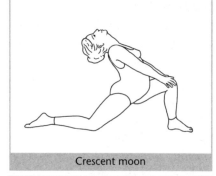

Crescent moon

Butterfly

(You may have practised this already in Baddha Konasana Supta.) Lie with your buttocks and feet against the wall. Keep the soles of your feet together and let your knees drop down to the sides. You can press down gently on your knees with your hands.

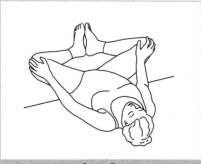

Butterfly

Spinal twist

Sit cross-legged on the floor. Place your opposite hand on your knee and the other hand on the floor behind you. Twist gently in the direction of the hand that's behind you. Repeat on the other side.

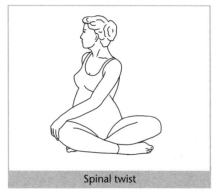

Spinal twist

Standing spinal twist

Stand with your legs crossed, then with arms outspread, twist in the direction of the front leg. Repeat on the other side.

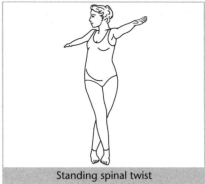

Standing spinal twist

The tree

Standing positions strengthen your legs and this one requires good balance too. Begin by putting the sole of your foot on the ankle bone of the other and with your hands in prayer position hold the pose. If you're an advanced student you can rest the sole of your foot on the inner thigh of the other leg.

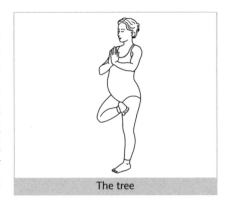

The tree

The child's pose

This position can be alternated with all the previous asanas. It opens the pelvic area, but you'll have to spread your knees wide apart to accommodate your growing belly.

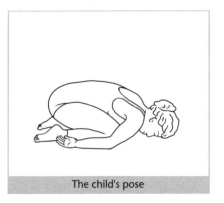

The child's pose

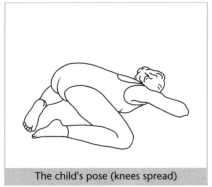

The child's pose (knees spread)

Modified abdominal corpse pose

Lying on your front, supporting your head on one or both arms, alternate the leg that is drawn up.

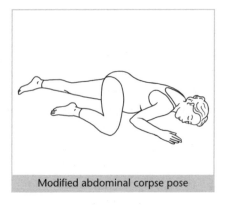

Modified abdominal corpse pose

The last two poses are both very good resting positions and are useful during the latter stages of your pregnancy when it's sometimes hard to find a comfortable position.

Belly dancing for an active birth

You might have a preconceived idea of a belly dancer as just one step removed from a burlesque show or stripper. However this dance form (also known as *raqs sharqi*), which originated in the Middle East, was first performed in ancient times when goddess worship was common. The performance is a celebration of life, fertility and the life-giving power of women, and the dance is also one of the earliest forms of preparation for childbirth. Belly dancing is now being taught as a safe and beneficial exercise option during pregnancy.

When practised on a regular basis it strengthens muscles and ligaments, improves circulation and leads to an improved awareness of abdominal and pelvic muscles that can give you much greater control over the birth process. It can also assist your baby's movement down the birth canal and can improve the efficiency of the uterine contractions. If you're a regular belly dancer you'll also make a speedier recovery after the birth. Classes are available in most areas—some are run under the auspices of maternity hospitals.

EXERCISING AFTER THE BIRTH

If you've been committed to regular exercise before and during your pregnancy, you'll probably be keen to get back to your old routine and may even be looking forward to the liberation of exercising without that big bump in your belly. But we've just got a few words of caution. Remember that you have just had a baby and in traditional societies women rarely return straight away to hard physical labour, even if they have been very active right up to the time of the birth. This is contrary to popular belief. The native woman who delivers her baby in the rice paddy and then returns immediately to back-breaking physical work is a mythical creature (or perhaps one who, unfortunately, has absolutely no other option).

Despite what you've been led to believe and despite your desire to be physically active again, your body, especially your uterus, pelvic floor and lower back, will take a little while to regain the shape and strength that it had before you conceived. Of course if you've been diligent with your exercise and stretching regimen, you'll be amazed at just how quickly and completely you get your old shape back, especially compared to women who have done no exercise at all.

Traditional wisdom recommends at least six weeks before you commence any serious aerobic activity, which will seem like an eternity if you're addicted to the endorphin hit that this type of exercise brings. Serious resistance or weight training should be on the back burner for about the same period of time. This gives your muscles and ligaments time to stabilise after the huge changes of pregnancy. Please don't think, as Jan did, that you know better. She waited (impatiently) for six weeks after the birth of her first son, but was back in training two weeks after the birth of her second and now suffers occasional lower back problems that stem from ignoring the potential instability of that area immediately after the birth. Of course, you can continue to stretch through the early weeks, and walking's fine, but at all times be guided by your body and do nothing that causes you any pain or discomfort.

Confidence and trust for a better birth

Confidence in your own ability to give birth is one of the foremost requirements for a better birth. Bringing a positive attitude to your labour and birth will keep your stress level down—and with it the fear and pain that so many Western women expect of labour. Although it's very natural to have some fears and anxieties, you need to balance these with trust in your own body. Which side of the see-saw you come down on can be a very delicate matter, and there are many factors which can tip the balance.

Imagine yourself as a circus acrobat in an act with two see-saws—one named 'FEAR/TRUST', the other called 'PAIN'. Your trusting self is on one side of the first see-saw, your stressed, anxious self is on the other. Your calm self comes down to earth, but your fearful self goes flying off into the air, turns several somersaults and comes down on the end of the second see-saw, which has your pain-free self on one side and your hurting self on the other. The extra weight of your stressed self sends your pain experience soaring. In turn, your hurting self comes down hard on the fear/stress side of the first see-saw and your previously grounded, calm self is off up in the air.

Pain is increased by many forms of stress. Physical tension is a direct cause, and this is exacerbated, in turn, by worry, uncertainty, loneliness, fear of the unknown, feelings of helplessness and passivity, lack of information and preparation, and the more physical problems such as fatigue and hunger. So in this chapter and the next we will look at some ways of overcoming any mental negativity you may be harbouring and, instead, ensuring you trust your body's ability to give birth to a healthy baby without the help of technology. We'll help you to feel confident, relaxed, rested, empowered, supported, informed, prepared and active.

YOUR EXPECTATIONS

Your expectations have a great deal to do with your labour and birth experience. Remember the ease with which women in traditional societies give birth? As well as their whole food diets and high levels of vigorous physical activity, something else about those women's lives was very different from ours. Since births in older cultures always occurred at home amongst family members and close friends, women had been present at births and had seen and heard what went on many times before they themselves became mothers.

In cultures where a family's living quarters were much more confined than they are today, a birth would have been an integral part of that family's life. It was not outside or apart from their routine day-to-day existence. It was never hidden away, so, from her very earliest years, a young girl would have observed her mother (and various aunts, sisters, cousins and girlfriends) while pregnant and during labour and birth. Since it was always the women of the community who attended a woman in labour, it is possible that by the time a young woman was ready to give birth to her own baby, she would have seen dozens of other women give birth to their children.

She would consider birth to be completely normal and natural. She would know that it hurt, but also that her body could deal with the pain, just as she had seen it dealt with many times. She would probably have seen a long labour, a difficult delivery, and a mother or baby who died, but overall her perception of the whole process would have been very different from the views of labour and birth which are almost universally held in Western society today.

If, like many Western women, you expect to feel overwhelming pain and be unable to cope, the probability is that you will resist the whole experience and hurt like hell. If, like women from traditional societies, you expect to have a strong, intense physical experience—a natural part of the process of life, which will probably shake you to your core—and are prepared for pain and ready to ride it, then you will come through it all intact and empowered.

It's probably *not* a good idea to imagine that your preparations will result in a pain-free birth. Most women experience some degree of pain, and you may feel inadequate during labour if you've expected to have none. Other women's fear of pain is such that they may choose an elective Caesarean to avoid it. The medicalisation of childbirth has led to the idea that pain is bad, and that drugs and surgery are a better choice. We've discussed some of the problems associated with these in Chapter 2, and rest our case. If you are confident that you can cope without these props, and welcome the chance to have a transformative experience, then you probably can and will.

BE PREPARED

Preparation is all-important in keeping you stress-free and confident. Studies show that educated women experience less pain in labour and childbirth, as do women who receive prenatal care and attend child-birth classes, and those whose husbands are supportive. So an important factor in having a better birth is finding out everything you can about the normal physiology of the birth process. As we've already explained, this was once easily achieved because giving birth was very much a normal part of life. But few women today have seen another woman in labour, let alone giving birth, now that this almost always happens in a hospital. In the absence of first hand experience, you must find other sources of information. Books and videos can help to fill the gaps, and talking to other women can be informative.

Books and videos

If you read widely you can learn what to expect in a normal birth and you can also find out a great deal more about all those obstetrical interventions that we have mentioned earlier. Of course it's important that your reading goes beyond the standard medical dogma—there are innumerable books, apart from ours, which question the routine medical management of birth and we have included a list in the Recommended Reading section.

Videos of women giving birth are probably even more valuable than books, since they can convey a more realistic picture of the actual experience. Make sure you watch some videos of women having a completely natural labour and birth—homebirth associations are usually a good source of these. You can make some very valuable comparisons if you also watch videos of women having a medically managed birth in a hospital setting.

Talking to new mothers

You should try to talk to as many women as possible who have given birth recently. However, some women might be reluctant conversationalists, especially if their labour and birth were not what they had been expecting, so you need to try a diplomatic approach. You could ask questions like these:

- *'Were you prepared for what happened?'*
- *'Were you comfortable in your surroundings?'*
- *'Did you feel as if you were in control?'*
- *'Was the information you received satisfactory?'*
- *'Were the reasons given for performing a particular procedure sufficient?'*
- *'Would you change anything next time around?'*

You can learn a great deal from the answers to these questions.

Women who have given birth without any intervention are usually much more willing to share their experiences. These women feel that they 'own' their birth and are usually eager to share their stories with others. Unfortunately, those women who have a completely natural labour and birth are still in a small minority, but it is important that you seek out some mothers who had their baby in a birthing centre or at home. Homebirth support groups most often have contacts who are happy to share their birth experiences with others. Invariably these groups publish newsletters and books that are full of personal birth accounts. Reading these can give you wonderful insight into the many different ways women labour and give birth. These stories can also let you see that a natural birth is something beautiful, something moving, something memorable, and ultimately something of great importance for all those present.

Childbirth education classes

Apart from reading books, watching videos and talking to other women, antenatal or childbirth education classes can be an excellent source of information. However, you should make careful inquiries before choosing a class. Some, particularly if they are run under the auspices of a maternity hospital, may be little more than preparation for a birth in hospital with all the usual interventions.

Therefore, before you sign up with any childbirth educator, you need to be sure that the classes are going to be of real benefit and that they will support you if you desire an active, intervention-free labour and birth. Your choice of a childbirth education class can determine whether you have the information you need to have a healthy and fulfiling childbirth experience. We have listed below some of the matters you'll need to canvass. (Our thanks to Lamaze International for permission to adapt their recommendations.)

- Make sure that your childbirth educator has undertaken comprehensive training.

- Find out how long she has been working as a childbirth educator and make sure that she regularly updates her knowledge.

- Ensure that she uses a variety of teaching strategies during each class. Since some individuals learn best by listening, while others may need to have visual cues and still others may need hands-on sessions, this will ensure that the needs of different types of learners will be met.

- Choose small, individualised classes. The ideal size is 6 to 10 couples (to a maximum of 12 couples). If the number of participants is very large it is unlikely that there will be much time for individual attention.

- The classes should consist of at least 12 hours instruction, with emphasis on practical skills supported by class discussion.

- Make sure that the curriculum supports birth as normal, natural and healthy, and empowers women to make informed choices about birth, breastfeeding and parenting.

※ The class content should include information about normal labour, birth and the early postpartum period, positioning to facilitate the normal progress of labour and birth, massage techniques to ease pain and enhance relaxation, other relaxation techniques, labour support, communication skills, information about medical procedures, and healthy lifestyle choices.

※ If the class is conducted in conjunction with a maternity hospital, make sure that all aspects of labour and birth will be discussed, not just how it is usually medically managed in the hospital setting.

※ Find out if the educator endorses your taking full personal responsibility for your birth experience, or whether she advocates following your obstetrician's orders.

※ Ask whether your educator will be available to answer your questions during the class and at other times during your pregnancy.

※ If you have an area of particular concern, make sure that this specific issue will be covered in the class.

※ Talk to some former students and get their feedback.

Even if you've diligently prepared for a better birth by amassing as much information as you can and you trust your body to labour and give birth successfully as women have for millennia, you may still have concerns about the processes and implications of birth and motherhood, and these may increase as you approach labour, especially if this is your first pregnancy.

FEARS AND ANXIETIES ARE NORMAL

It's normal and natural to be like this—you're not the first expectant mother to feel this way. Let's look at some of the anxieties that may be plaguing you and try to dispel them.

Emotional fluctuations

Not only is this a major and transformative life event that is approaching (and fast!), but your high level of circulating hormones makes this a time of increased sensitivity. This may manifest as a heightening of your psychic senses, of your awareness of the daily miracles of life and nature, alternating with increased levels of anxiety. These emotional fluctuations are a common experience towards the end of pregnancy and there is no need to add to your emotional load by feeling guilty or concerned about them. Any tendency to be more instinctive in your reactions, and to have a less intellectual or rational response to events or other people is a natural part of this stage of pregnancy— so enjoy it! You will return to your 'normal' self in due course—for good or bad.

'Irrational' concerns

Thoughts such as *'How will this great big lump ever get out through my vagina?'* will surface. It will—if your zinc levels are good your ligaments and skin will stretch easily and, despite the scaremongering that you may be exposed to, most babies are an appropriate size for their mother's pelvis. These thoughts and concerns are likely to be more intense if this is your first baby, or if you have little familiarity with others' births. You may find it helpful to voice your anxieties with your partner, your midwife or doctor, your childbirth educator, or a friend. This can stop the fears becoming obsessive. Nobody will think it strange for you to have concerns, and your professional caregivers will have experience in offering support at this time.

Fear of letting go

For many women, especially those used to exerting a high level of self-determination in their affairs, the inevitability of the approaching birth and their apparent loss of control over events can be frightening. It's true, there's no stopping things now. This baby has got to be born, but there are many ways in which you can make this a joyous and positive experience. This may make you feel more as if you are 'back in the driver's seat', if that's where you feel comfortable. For others, relinquishing control at this time and surrendering to the natural unfolding can also be a comfort. Some women fear other, more physical, lapses in control, such as having their waters break in public, urinating, vomiting or defecating during labour, or the loss of emotional control. We'd like to reassure you that if this does happen, it's unlikely that it will bother you. In fact you'll *need* to lose control as giving birth is all about letting yourself ride the strong waves of energy that emanate from your mind and body. It's also unlikely to bother those around you, who will be much more concerned with the safe birth of your baby. Your midwife or doctor has seen it all before, while your partner will be in awe of the whole experience and full of an overwhelming admiration for you.

Fear of pain or medical intervention

Other normal fears are to do with your capacity to cope with the pain of birth or of interventions such as forceps, Caesareans and episiotomies. Far from fearing the experience of pain and seeking to avoid it, you may find that embracing it, or observing it during labour and birth, can ensure your experience is a positive one. Develop an interest in your sensations, feel with your mind their location, their intensity, their rhythms and patterns, how they change as you breathe, move and adopt different positions. Go deep within yourself and experience the pain from the inside, instead of feeling like a victim. Flow with it, experience it as a transforming experience that is bigger than you, but not hostile to you.

You can attach these sensations to a particular visualisation to help you flow with the experience, or adopt a different approach by going 'somewhere else' and using visualisation techniques to remove yourself from the pain; allowing it its own reality, but focusing your mind elsewhere. Breathing techniques are also an effective way of releasing endorphins, nature's own pain killers. We'll look at some ideas for visualisations, breathing techniques and other ways of coping with pain in the next chapter.

However, just as women have been celebrating the birthing process all through time, there have also been those who have suffered. If you end up choosing pain relief or a medical option, there is no need to feel you have failed. Each birth is its own justification, each child a miracle to be wondered at. The method of delivery is just that, a way of getting a child into the world. The trick is to keep your mind open to all possibilities, especially that of a good experience. If you don't get caught up in a fixed idea of how your birth will be, you increase the chances of responding naturally and appropriately to whatever happens.

Other fears and anxieties during the birth

You may well be too preoccupied with the physical process of giving birth to worry about anything at all! But since staying relaxed is important to ensure an easy labour, if may be helpful to be forewarned of some possible feelings.

If you are giving birth in a hospital, your first fear may be of unfamiliar surroundings, equipment and personnel. Even if you don't expect to end up in hospital, you may find it helpful to visit a labour ward in advance to 'acclimatise' yourself, and ensure that you can have your support people with you through the labour.

Lack of privacy in a hospital environment may also be a cause for concern, and also the hospital's expectations of your behaviour (some labour wards still ask you to be 'quiet' so as not to disturb other mothers). These issues are less likely to be a problem if you have chosen your hospital well, and discussed its policies.

Giving birth at home is more likely to be a supportive and relaxing experience, as long as you have confidence in your carers and support people. If being at home is going to increase your anxiety about things going wrong, then this may not be the best choice for you. A birthing centre may be a good compromise, providing an informal environment with easy access to the labour ward.

Nearly all labouring mothers reach a state when they wonder if they have the strength or reserves to continue. This, accompanied by the knowledge that you really have no choice (other than a Caesarean), can lead to panic. If you know in advance that you may feel like this, you can call on your innate and learnt coping mechanisms, and be assured that your second (or third or fourth!) wind will kick in. The physical strength to push may sometimes seem lacking, but the encouragement of your carers and supporters will get you through. Remember that few labours last longer than 24 hours (usually many fewer if you do all the right things before conception and during your pregnancy), and nearly all mothers happily do it all over again!

If the labour is long, and fatigue sets in, your emotions may simply boil over. You may start to feel anger or resentment towards your midwife or doctor (for not giving you relief), your partner (for getting you into this in the first place), your unborn baby (for causing you pain) and the gods and goddesses (for allowing life to hold such challenges). If you, and everyone else, are aware that this may happen, there is no need for it to overwhelm you or for them to take it personally or react badly (although we can't answer for the gods and goddesses!).

Don't be afraid to express your needs

It's really helpful to be sufficiently in contact with your physical and emotional feelings to be able to identify and express your needs during labour and birth. Being sufficiently relaxed to be able to focus your mind on the cascade of sensations you are experiencing is an important part of ensuring that these needs are recognised and met, but your capacity to ask for and receive help and communicate your needs clearly is also essential if you are to have a good experience. Your support people and carers are only too keen to give you whatever help they can, but may not know how to be most effective unless you tell them. Don't worry if your demands come out in a vigorous or abrupt fashion—the whole experience of birth is vigorous, primal and awe-inspiring for everyone present, and you don't have to be polite or concerned about others' feelings. Everyone present has, as their major aim, the safe birth of your child, and your wellbeing. Let them help you—they need to feel of use.

Fears for your unborn baby

All mothers have moments of panic when they think their baby has stopped moving, or is lurching about excessively. If you've decided to trust your body and forgo the high-tech procedures during your pregnancy, you can still be reassured that all is progressing well. Babies, just like anyone else, have times of greater and lesser activity, and you should just remind yourself that your anxiety is normal. Let the fears pass through you and over you and watch them leave. Most mothers have dreams of giving birth to monsters, or kittens, but the chances of there being anything wrong with your baby are remote, and even less likely if you have paid attention to your health before and during pregnancy. However, if your concerns persist, talk to your midwife (or doctor) and let her decide whether there's really anything to worry about.

She will already be checking your blood pressure and urine routinely. Abdominal palpation, or manual feeling of your belly, can be performed to assess the size and position of your baby and a stethoscope can detect the foetal heartbeat from about 24 weeks.

You should also be aware (and you will be if you've read our earlier books) that if any problems arise during your pregnancy, there is a great deal that you can do to help in their management. Natural remedies such as herbs and nutritional supplements, meditation, visualisation, acupuncture, chiropractic adjustment, aromatherapy and massage can all be used effectively (see Chapters 7 and 9). (If your baby stops moving altogether, then you must seek immediate help.)

Fear of approaching motherhood

You may also be anxious about approaching motherhood. You may dream that you go shopping and leave your baby behind at the cash register! Or, if this is not your first child, your fears may focus on the concern that this baby will increase your workload unbelievably, or interfere with your precious relationships with your existing children, or your partner. If you are a working mother, you may worry that you will be unable to fulfil your job commitments. Some mothers-to-be, especially those with many children, those having their first baby, or those lacking support in their relationship, may have fears that their partner will leave them alone to cope with their expanding family. All we can say is that you should voice these concerns, share them with friends and family, but remember that life unfolds in unexpected ways, and you will probably surprise yourself at how well you manage all of these aspects of motherhood. The great joy and euphoria accompanying the birth of a baby will give you unexpected strength and good humour.

Fears for your relationship with your partner

Increasing fatigue late in pregnancy can lead to an inability to concentrate, to impatience with those close to you, general irritability and lack of libido. You may become depressed about the size and appearance of your body, about your inability to get physically comfortable, to exercise, to find clothes that fit and about the difficulty of having good sex. Cuddles and kisses can be very comforting, but you may be worried about the effect of all of this on your partner.

If you can, try talking this through. Chances are your fears are ungrounded, and just part of general feelings of vulnerability. Instead, enjoy! Let yourself be pampered by your partner (and others), revel in the attention you command, and accept *all* offers of help. Especially, don't let yourself get caught up with anxiety that you won't live up to others' expectations of you (or your own of yourself). Try not to have any expectations. Birth and motherhood are never as expected, and you will find that it all comes quite naturally, taken one day at a time.

You should recognise, however, that most fathers-to-be also have anxieties, especially the first time around. Your partner may feel unable to express these, especially to you, whom he considers to have enough worries of your own and, in fact, be in need of his support and comfort.

One of his main concerns may centre around his ability to provide this succour, both before and during the birth, and also afterwards when the new baby makes demands on time and finances. But fathers, like mothers, are primarily concerned that their baby will be healthy, that the labour will go well and that their partner will cope with the demands of giving birth.

His anxieties about his own role will start with the need to call the midwife in time for a home birth, or get you to the hospital in time. He may also be worried that he will be elsewhere, and miss the birth altogether. As well as being concerned that you might not cope well with the demands of giving birth, he may also fear that the blood and guts will be too much for him, that he will panic, and that he won't do the right things at the right time. After all, he will have no contractions to focus his mind and energies! Many fathers feel powerless during labour, and it's important that your partner, if he is to be present, is well coached in how he can be an 'active' participant, and not just a spectator. Of course, it's also up to you to let him know what he can do for you at different stages. If he is to attend the birth, then you will probably have attended pre-natal classes together, but some dads don't feel comfortable about attending the birth, and some mums prefer an all-women affair. You need to know each other's feelings about this well ahead of time. If he is not going to be present at the birth, then you'll need to work out a way for him to be there as soon as possible afterwards, so you can all bond as a family, and he can hold and acknowledge his child right away.

Of course, in some situations a child is born outside a relationship, or to one in which the father is not committed to the mother, or to raising a child. If this is clear from the start you will have to find other support systems. But even in an on-going and apparently successful relationship, an imminent birth can bring up all sorts of questions for the father, such as *'Do I really want to be a father?'* and *'Do I really want to stay in this relationship forever?'* These are very normal concerns, because having a baby will bring about dramatic changes in the best of relationships. Recognising this, and being ready to acknowledge and discuss your partner's concerns, while feeling free to express your own, will usually stand you (and your relationship) in good stead.

STAYING RESTED AND STRESS FREE

As we've seen, physical fatigue can increase your emotional vulnerability and stress levels, and it is important to have plenty of sleep, especially as labour can start at any time of the day or night, and quite commonly in the early hours of the morning. You will need all your energy and strength if you're to experience a better birth, and should be well rested. Take an afternoon nap whenever possible, and get to bed early. Your sleep may be disturbed by the need to urinate, and by the difficulty of finding a comfortable position for your increasing bulk. The famous 'nesting instinct' may have you cleaning at all hours cupboards that have stayed comfortably grubby for years, scrubbing saucepans that you haven't used in a decade and sorting through boxes of papers that have no relevance to your child's birth. While this is a natural preparation for the addition to your family, remember that rest is more important and your baby couldn't give a hoot whether the kitchen is tidy or whether the nursery is decorated with soft toys. All he wants is to be close to you, warm and fed. It's particularly unhelpful to add to your stress by doing any decorating at this time, especially as many paints and solvents release toxic fumes.

Just pay attention to your preparations, make your birth plan (see Chapter 8) and allow yourself to get excited. You may well feel by now that it's time for a change. Pregnancy is reaching its end and you're on the brink of a whole new, wonderful, transforming experience—that of becoming a mother. Even if you're already a mother, each child brings the opportunity all over again, and each child touches a different part of you.

ACKNOWLEDGING CHANGE

Some women feel the need at this time for some kind of ritual or rite of passage. This could be a spiritual or religious ceremony, performed with friends and family present, or alone with just your unborn baby as witness. It could involve contact with nature. You might like to plant a tree, or set up a little 'altar' to motherhood, womanhood and fertility.

The most common social event will be a baby 'shower' with gifts offered by female relatives and friends. This is often the time when the 'elders' of your community, and those who've already had children, offer advice. We'd like to offer you some, too. Don't listen to any negative stories. Just politely decline and assert your right not to be distressed. All the advice in the world is unimportant compared to your own innate and instinctive knowledge about birth and motherhood. Anxieties and fears just come between you and your inner voice. Staying calm, relaxed and confident in your own abilities is the best way to contact your needs and strengths.

You should also give yourself permission to make your own mistakes. Many parents-to-be are so determined not to make the mistakes their parents made, they lose sight of the best way to deal with a new and different situation. Freeing yourself to make your own mistakes is best achieved by forgiving your own parents theirs. All parents are humans too; there is no such thing as a perfect parent.

If your emotional state becomes too fraught to contemplate a joyful ritual, all you may need is a really good cry! Weeping is a good way of letting go of anxiety. Shed some tears with someone you love and trust, or simply offer up your fears to the great goddess inherent in us all.

Acknowledging your fears and anxieties, examining your expectations, acquiring knowledge and staying rested are all important ways to build your confidence and trust that your body is designed to give birth to babies.

Coping with stress and pain for a better birth

Well, you may say, it's all very fine telling me about all the fears and anxieties I'm entitled to, but how shall I best manage them? In this chapter we'll try to give you some ideas for coping with the stresses both before and during childbirth.

BREATHING TECHNIQUES

One thing you may well learn at your antenatal classes, or with your midwife, is the breathing technique to use while giving birth. But breathing is also an excellent way to relax, so we'll look at that first. You'll be able to use this technique during pregnancy as well as between contractions during labour.

Breathing to relax

The simplest way to relax using breathing is to direct your breath to each part of your body in turn, tensing that part as you inhale, then relaxing as you exhale—and becoming aware of how different that body part feels as it relaxes. Here's how to proceed.

- First, sit or lie comfortably, your legs uncrossed, your back and head supported, your eyes closed. Start to breathe easily and rhythmically.

- Then practise a deep inhalation and exhalation. Place your hand on your belly and feel it rise off your uterus as you draw the breath deep down inside. When you exhale, keep letting go of the breath even when you think it is all gone.

- Now, as you inhale, tighten all your muscles, all over your body. Form your hands into fists, screw your face up into a frown, clench your jaw and your buttocks, pull your shoulders up and your tummy in, tighten your calves, thighs, feet, arms and back muscles and feel your hair rise as your scalp tightens.

- Then, as you exhale, let all of these muscles go. Feel your facial muscles relax into a gentle smile, your hands, feet, arms and legs release, your shoulders drop, your back and buttocks relax and your tummy resemble a laughing Buddha statue.

- Now, with each breath, and starting with your toes, move up your body one part at a time, tensing on the in-breath, and relaxing and letting go on the out-breath. Let that part of your body feel heavy, focus on the contact between it and the chair, bed or floor, and feel warmth flood through it.

- When you've reached your scalp, just lie or sit comfortably for a while with easy, rhythmic breathing, feeling calm and quiet, and focusing on the breath entering and leaving your body.

- Finish this activity by sending one deep breath to your mind to clear your thoughts, igniting there a golden glow. The next breath goes to your heart to bring joy and courage, and igniting another golden glow. A third, and final, breath goes to your womb and your baby, taking your love and comfort, and surrounding the area with yet another golden glow. Then, as you breathe easily and rhythmically, feel these glowing centres of energy expand, until they join and fill your whole body with strong, calm energy, ready for whatever lies ahead.

If you practise this technique during pregnancy and become familiar with its use, you'll be able to use it confidently in labour between contractions.

Breathing for contractions

There are two different schools of thought about how to breathe through contractions. The Lamaze method teaches a deep breath at the start of a contraction, followed by increasingly rapid and shallow breaths as the contraction peaks, releasing with another deep breath at the end of the contraction. Women who use this method find centering the breathing in their chest or mouth distracts them from the pain of the contraction, and helps them to feel more in control. The Bradley method advocates keeping the breathing deep all through the contraction, encouraging you to focus deep down within your body, in your belly. This may help you to stay more relaxed, and avoids the risk of hyperventilation. Your antenatal caregiver may have their own preference, but you may find that learning all the different types of breathing can give you a wider repertoire of coping tools.

Endorphins, the body's natural painkillers, are increased through both deep and rapid breathing, and give you the power to dissolve pain as you feel it approach, as well as staying centred and relaxed.

Many mothers use the analogy of surfing when talking about breathing through contractions: feeling the pain pulling on you like the undertow before a wave, feeling it swell as the contraction begins, catching the crest with your breath and surfing on, with the wave, to the safe beach. As in surfing, the timing of the breath is the key: the deep, cleansing inhalation starting as the contraction begins, deep or rapid breathing continuing as you surf the wave, and the final deep exhalation helping you to ride the wave to shore. As you exhale, you will find it easier to relax and release all tensions, accepting the contraction and surrendering to its power. Both the contraction and your breath have their own rhythms, and when these synchronise you will feel confident that you can ride the waves. It's most important not to hold your breath, which is a common response to pain, anxiety and tension, but just increases the problem. Rhythmic breathing keeps you in control, and ensures sufficient oxygen for you and your baby. The most relaxing time is on the exhalation, and you may find it helpful to keep your mouth and jaw soft and open during the out breath, associating this with a soft, open cervix. As there is an unconscious neuromuscular connection between the vagina and the mouth, this association is quite real.

Let's look now at the different ways of breathing.

For *deep breathing*, practise keeping your hand on your belly, which should expand as you inhale, your hand rising. Your support person should be able to feel this expansion right down in your lower back, as you draw the breath deep down inside to your belly. It's like a deep yawn, and you should try and keep your shoulders relaxed. This is appropriate for the gentle contractions of the early first stage of labour, and may be your preferred way to deal with the more intense contractions of late first stage.

For *light breathing*, practise keeping your hand on your upper chest, which should expand as you inhale, only using the upper part of your lungs. Your support person can feel this in your upper back and shoulders. Keep your mouth slightly open and take short, sharp breaths. These may get lighter and shallower and centred higher and higher in your chest, and eventually only in your mouth, which avoids the hyperventilation that can result from shallow chest breathing. This may be your preferred way of dealing with contractions as they increase in intensity, as it releases the pressure on your abdomen. Light breathing will automatically be more rapid than deep breathing.

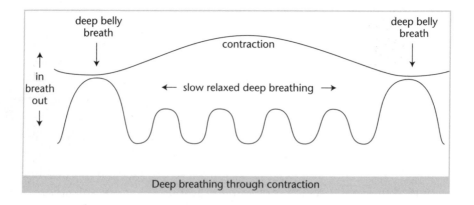

Deep breathing through contraction

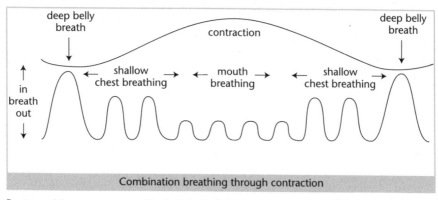

Combination breathing through contraction

In transition, you may find it helpful to *pant* or *blow*. This can help to stop you pushing (sometimes called bearing down) before the cervix is fully dilated, as it's physically impossible to push at the same time. If this breathing is focused in your mouth rather than your chest, it will help to avoid hyperventilation, which can make you feel light-headed, and cause your hands and feet to go numb and tense into a claw-like position. This is not good for your baby, and you should cover your mouth and nose with your hand (or your supporter's), re-breathing your own air, or use a paper bag to achieve the same effect. Another way to avoid hyperventilation is to hold your breath for five seconds after each ten pants, but take care—if you hold your breath for more than six or seven seconds, the oxygen supply to your baby is reduced. It's helpful to use rhythmic sets of three breaths—two pants followed by a blow, or two blows followed by a pant.

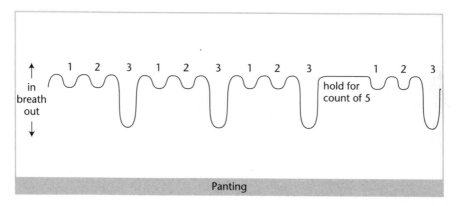

Panting

In the second stage of labour, deep breathing will help you to push. Take a deep breath, and either push as you hold the breath, and then exhale at the end, or push as you exhale. The choice may depend on whether you feel like pushing, or just 'opening up', which may be easier during exhalation. This feeling can be quite sensual, with some women comparing giving birth to orgasm. Birth is, after all, the completion of the sexual cycle for women, following the desire, conception, and pregnancy—all part of nature's plan.

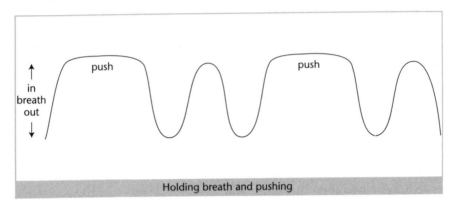

Holding breath and pushing

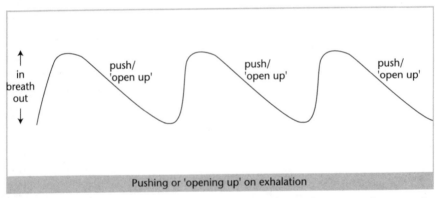

Pushing or 'opening up' on exhalation

With any of these techniques, you may find it helps to make sounds as you exhale. A sighing sound may help you feel that you are releasing tension, and groaning or moaning sounds from deep down in your belly trigger endorphin production. Although high-pitched screaming is counter-productive, don't be afraid to yell, roar, shout and be thoroughly noisy and uninhibited if this is what you need to do.

All these techniques will need to be practised well before your due date, and you need to have a good understanding with your midwife or doctor so that you are not at cross-purposes. She may have a preferred method, but it all gets back to your expectations and staying open-minded. There is no one way that is best, and you may find you draw on different techniques at different times. If you stay relaxed and focused on your body's demands, this won't be confusing, merely intuitive and natural. Don't get hung up on a particular method, just practise the different types of breathing, learn how they feel, what they do for you (to release abdominal pressure—light breaths, or to increase it—deep breaths), and do what seems to help most. Breathing, like the adoption of different positions for giving birth, is pretty instinctive.

MEDITATION/VISUALISATION/ AFFIRMATION

Meditation, visualisations and affirmations can be used to help you relax, both during your pregnancy and when you're in labour. They can help you enter the pain and work with it, or take your mind somewhere else, letting your body handle the pain in its own way. You might, for example, visualise your cervix opening up and your baby's head coming through, or you might imagine your cervix as a flower opening like the time-lapse photography featured in nature programs. Alternatively, you might visualise the waves and surfing that we suggested earlier as an analogy for your contractions. Water is a common theme in women's birthing images; it is powerful and supportive at the same time, and swells and surges in the same way as your body's sensations. If you want to distract your mind from your body, you could imagine yourself in a favourite place.

One of the easiest ways to stay focused and calm is to use a mantra or an affirmation. You may have a favourite single-word mantra that you have become accustomed to in previous meditation sessions, or you may want to choose something that is meaningful for you right now, such as 'let go', 'release' or 'open up'. We'd like to give you some other suggestions for affirmations to use in the later stages of pregnancy, or during the birth.

- 'I have innate knowledge for birth and motherhood.'
- 'I embrace the intensity of birth.'
- 'The birth of my baby is a miracle of life.'
- 'I embrace the pain of birth as part of my initiation into motherhood.'
- 'I will reach down inside myself and feel my body's needs.'
- 'I will make my needs clear to others.'

- *'I will accept the help I need.'*
- *'I am open to my best possible birth.'*
- *'However my baby comes into this world, it's his own path.'*
- *'I trust in my body's ability to give birth naturally.'*
- *'I trust my caregivers to help me make the best possible decisions.'*
- *'I trust in my strength.'*
- *'I trust in my ability to stay relaxed and positive throughout my baby's birth.'*
- *'I welcome the birth of my child.'*

HYPNOTHERAPY

Another way to create a relaxed and positive attitude during birth is through hypnotherapy or auto-suggestion. This can best be achieved by working with a clinical hypnotherapist in the last six weeks or so of your pregnancy. When you are in a deeply relaxed state (hypnotised) your subconscious is amenable to positive ideas. Suggestions can then be made that you will stay relaxed and positive during labour, make the best use of your learned and innate knowledge, be able to identify your needs, express them to others and receive help, and be able to flow with the contractions and stay on top of the pain. Your hypnotherapist may suggest to you that when a certain event happens you will react in a particular, positive way, or may teach you self-hypnosis so you can do this for yourself. You may also find it helpful to have a tape made of the suggestions, so you can listen to it as you approach, or even during, the birth.

Hypnotherapy has a proven successful track record with childbirth, though it's best to choose a practitioner who has experience in this particular field. One study showed that hypnosis reduced labour time by 98 minutes in first-time mothers, and by 40 minutes in mothers who had given birth before, compared to the control group. In this study, the mothers undergoing hypnosis also experienced greater satisfaction with the birth.

In another study, comparison was made between two groups of mothers who had babies presenting in the breech position (bottom down) between the thirty-seventh and fortieth weeks of pregnancy. The babies in the group receiving hypnotherapy turned satisfactorily into the head down position at twice the rate of those in the control group. The focus in this study was on releasing the emotional turmoil that these mothers commonly felt to be associated with the breech position.

Yet another study showed that women using hypnotherapy used 11.4 per cent fewer epidurals than those in the control group, and 17.9 per cent fewer than another group of low-risk women. They also had 18.5 per cent fewer drips and 15.9 per cent fewer episiotomies than the women in the control and low-risk groups, and the second stage of labour was slightly shorter.

TOUCHIE-FEELIES

Relaxation will always be most effective if the techniques used focus on relieving both mental and physical stress. While mental relaxation (such as affirmations, visualisation and hypnotherapy) will also soothe physical tensions, the reverse is also true, and a body-centred approach to stress reduction is particularly appropriate during the extremely physically demanding experience of childbirth.

Touch

Touch is a marvellous tool for relaxation, and can be employed by anyone with whom you feel comfortable. It can be used in late pregnancy or during labour by your partner, support people, friends and even your children, and doesn't require any massage skills, though it'll probably work better during labour if you've practised it during the previous weeks. Here are some ideas.

- Ask your partner/friend/support person to touch or stroke lightly any area where you feel tension. Feel the tension flow from your body, through their hand and away.

- Ask if they can tell where tension is accumulating (e.g. your shoulders may be hunched, your face screwed up), and actively seek out these areas to touch or stroke. This will be helpful when you are distracted by intense contractions.

- Ask them if they can imagine that they are a channel for your tension release (they may like to imagine it flowing right through them and down into the floor).

- Another version of touch relaxation is to tense each body part in turn, as described above in the section on breathing for relaxation, and then have someone touch that body part to release it. This is a helpful way to practise touch relaxation in the last weeks of your pregnancy, so you associate the touch or stroke with a release of tension.

Not every woman wants to be touched during labour, and some of you may not have anyone with whom you feel sufficiently physically intimate to be comfortable using this approach. However, if you do, it's likely that a massage will be even more deeply appreciated than simple touch.

Massage

Many studies have confirmed what we knew all along—massage is an excellent way to reduce stress. One study looked at the effect of massage on a group of depressed, adolescent expectant mothers, and found positive changes in behaviour, including reduced anxiety and pulse rate, and also in levels of cortisol, a stress hormone. In another study, when massage was used as well as breathing techniques during late pregnancy and labour, there was a measurable decrease in anxiety, depression and pain, a shorter labour and hospital stay, and less postnatal depression. So get in there and learn how! (or choose support people who can help).

Most people find it hugely relaxing and comforting to have their **neck, shoulders, head** and **face** massaged or stroked. On the shoulders you can use quite strong pressure, with fingers, thumbs and the heel of your hand, on the neck it's best to use the fingers and thumbs, pulling the muscle away from the spine, or stroking up towards the skull. Lots of tension collects in the scalp, and the action here should be very similar to that used when washing the hair—you can even tug gently on handfuls of hair to stimulate the scalp. Only light pressure, either stroking or firm but light movements, should be used on the face. Movements should be either circular or away from the centre (when you tense, you usually screw everything up towards the middle). Look at yourself frowning, scowling and with pursed lips, and you'll see what we mean. Light touch over the eyelids can be helpful to release tension in tired eyes.

Firm massage of the **lower back** can be extremely helpful in releasing the pain of contractions, which often results in backache. Get your helper to find the base of your spine, between your buttocks, and massage firmly in a circular motion, using the heel of the hand, on either side of the spine. The more intense the pain (i.e. during contractions), the firmer the counter pressure should be.

Your **belly** could probably do with some light massage too—you can also do this for yourself. A very good massage for releasing tension in this area is one done in time with your inhalations and exhalations. You can use either a circular motion, up on the right side of the body as you breathe in and down on the left as you breathe out (following the ascending and descending colons), or use a simple downward stroke from the solar plexus to the pubic bone on each out breath. The touch should be light but firm, using the whole hand (see Diagram 1). You can also keep up a continuous movement that includes the upper **thighs** (see Diagram 2).

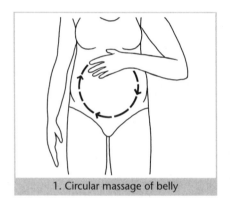

1. Circular massage of belly

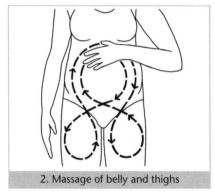

2. Massage of belly and thighs

While you're paying attention to the front of your body, a little **nipple** stimulation (by your partner, perhaps) can help the uterus to contract, and speed up the labour. One study showed that self-massage of the breasts from the thirty-ninth week of pregnancy reduced the incidence of significantly postmature births by 70 per cent.

When massaging the **limbs**, which may feel tired and aching, always stroke towards the heart. That brings us to two of the most useful areas for massage, the **hands** and **feet**. Pulling on fingers and toes, and rubbing between them, can be very relaxing. When rubbing the palms and soles, it's best to press with the thumbs in different spots and work from the centre to the edges. Be firm, especially with the feet, where a light touch can be very ticklish. If you can't suppress the tickle, a firm slapping action on the soles can help. Both the hands and the feet have special pressure points that can be used to great effect.

Reflexology

Reflexology has been shown in an English study to assist greatly in easing childbirth. Treatments that are started at any time from the twentieth week of pregnancy seem to lead to shorter, easier labours and there are also points that can be used during labour.

There is a theory that, traditionally, women have held onto bedposts during labour for the good reason that this affects helpful pressure points on the palms and fingers. A specific way to stimulate these points and hasten a sluggish labour is to hold a strong comb in each hand, pressing on the points at the base and tip of each finger, and the tip of the thumb.

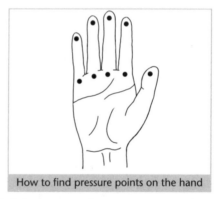

How to find pressure points on the hand

There are also helpful areas and points on the feet. Try rubbing the areas for the solar plexus (for anxiety and fear—this can help if you have palpitations), the lungs (to help keep breathing steady and rhythmic, and avoid hyperventilation) and the heart (for palpitations). There is also a special 'labour' point at the base of the second and third toes—see the diagrams page 279 to help you find the right spots. Note that there are reflex areas for the lungs on both the top and base of each foot.

Other pressure points

There are pressure points on other areas of the body that can be stimulated during a massage in late pregnancy or labour to trigger the release of stress and muscular tension. It is appropriate to use 'calming pressure' by caressing the point with the palm of your hand, or by gently stroking for about two minutes.

Pericardium 6: This point is three finger-widths up from the wrist crease on the inside of your arm, between the two tendons (third finger finds the spot). It should be calmed and can help you to sleep. (This point should *not* be used in the fourth month of pregnancy).

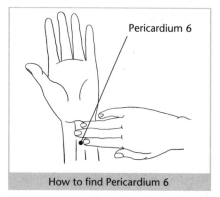

How to find Pericardium 6

Stomach 45: This point can also help you to sleep as well as calm you. You'll find it on the bottom outer corner of the nail bed of the second toe, on the side nearest to the third toe. It should *not* be used in the sixth month of pregnancy.

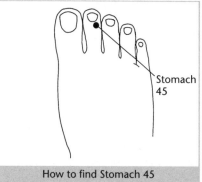

How to find Stomach 45

Acupressure to specific points can also ease the pain of giving birth, and for this you may want to use a firmer pressure with thumb or forefinger, in a circular anti-clockwise motion, or a pumping action, in and out, on the point. The pressure can initially be applied fairly deeply, and then brought up to the surface. This is called 'dispersing' the energy, which has become blocked at the point, causing a problem.

Take care to keep the area as relaxed as possible, and increase the pressure gradually each time you visit the point, so there is not a tensing reaction. Try these two points for pain relief during labour (*not during pregnancy*):

Bladder 32: This point can be found on the lower back, in the second groove in the sacrum, three finger-widths on either side of the spine. DO NOT USE THIS POINT DURING PREGNANCY.

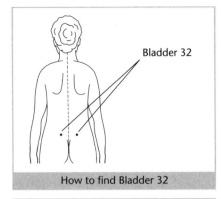

How to find Bladder 32

Spleen 6: This point can be found four finger-widths (the fourth finger finds the spot) above the interior ankle bone, in the small hollow just behind the tibia. DO NOT USE THIS POINT DURING PREGNANCY.

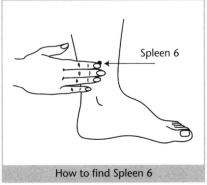

How to find Spleen 6

It's also useful, during a massage, to pay particular attention to the whole of the sacrum, especially the tip.

During acupuncture, when needles are used instead of pressure, greater stimulation of the points can be achieved. For this you need to have a qualified acupuncturist attending your birth, who may also stimulate the points with heat from a glowing stick of compressed *Mugwort* herb, called 'Moxa'. Acupuncture can not only relieve pain and stress, but also strengthen contractions and shorten the duration of labour. Studies show that these benefits can be quite substantial, and that women receiving acupuncture during labour generally report feeling greater calm and a sense of wellbeing and control over their own labour and delivery. (See Appendix 1 for more on how to use acupressure.)

Aromatherapy

If you incorporate essential oils in a massage, you can make it much more effective. The best oil for pain relief is *Clary Sage*, which also has both sedative and vitalising effects (sedating anxieties as well as increasing healthy energy). Other oils which are helpful when you are in pain are *Rose* (which can also relieve feelings of vulnerability and sadness), *Jasmine* (which is also uplifting and soothing) and *Ylang Ylang* (which has a sedating action). These oils can be mixed together in a massage oil base. (Try sweet almond or grapeseed oil in the ratio of one drop of essential oil to each 2 mL of base oil. Or try vitamin E cream with one drop of oil required for each 4 g of cream.) Use a few drops of each oil, from one drop to fifteen, depending on your preference. These fragrances are particularly helpful if used on the back and abdomen, which are the centres of pain. (If you know of a particular point that will benefit from a direct application, you can use one drop of the undiluted oil there.) If you have no-one to massage you, or don't feel like being touched, you could try a towel soaked in hot water to which the oils have been added. Wring out all excess moisture and place it over the painful area. Essential oils can also be used in oil burners and baths, as we'll describe shortly.

Osteopathy and chiropractic

In one study in the US, it was demonstrated that regular osteopathic treatments during pregnancy can significantly reduce both foetal and maternal fatalities as well as the incidence of difficult labours. Both osteopathy and chiropractic have been shown to be safe for both mother and unborn child, and regular spinal and soft tissue manipulation during pregnancy has also been shown to result in a much lower incidence of back pain in the later stages of pregnancy and during childbirth.

Be wary, however (especially if seeing a chiropractor), of any use of X-ray, which should be completely avoided during pregnancy (and during the preconception period) since ionising radiation has an adverse effect on cells with a rapid rate of division (such as those in eggs, sperm and a growing foetus).

SETTING THE SCENE

We've already mentioned how comforting familiar surroundings can be, and how strange places can make you anxious and tense. There are lots of things you can bring to your birthing environment to make it more relaxing and help you have a better birth.

Music

Not everyone finds music helpful, and some women experience it as an unwelcome distraction, but it's worth having your favourite CDs and tapes around as several studies have shown that music can help women to relax and focus their attention, energy and motivation on the task of giving birth. Some recordings are made specifically for relaxation and are designed to slow the heartbeat, regulate breathing and calm the mind. Alternatively, you may prefer classical or sacred music. You might even find a gallop or a polka (try Strauss!) helps you to feel more energetic when your energy lags. Remember your baby can hear the music too—you may have felt your child 'dancing' in your womb during pregnancy.

Heaven-scent

Essential oils (or incense) can generate fragrances to help calm or energise you, and can also be used to disinfect the labour room. All you need is a few drops in a water-based or electric burner, in a bowl of warm water, or on a hot, wet towel. *Lavender*, *Lemon* and *Bergamot* are antiseptic, as is *Tea-tree*, and these can be blended together. *Lavender*, *Ylang Ylang*, *Geranium*, *Chamomile*, *Mandarin*, *Sandalwood*, *Neroli*, *Jasmine* and *Rose* will help you to stay calm and relaxed, both before and during your labour.

WATER AND HEAT

You may find that water helps you to cope with the pain of contractions. If it's possible, you could get into a deep warm bath, and when you're suspended in the water, imagine your body opening up completely. Water has soothing, relaxing properties and lots of women choose to stay in the bath throughout their labour. Studies show that warm water causes the cervix to dilate twice as fast, so the first stage of labour is significantly shortened. (However, if your labour is not properly established, water can cause it to stop completely.) Special birth pools are available for hire, and many maternity units offer women the option of labouring and birthing in such a pool. If you don't have access to a bath or birth pool, get a plastic stool or chair, put it under the shower and have a good long soak.

In a bath, you can use the same oils that we've suggested for your oil-burner. You will need a dispersing base so that the oil doesn't collect in droplets on the top of the bath water. You can buy fragrance free, dispersing bath oil and add your own preferred aromas. You'll only need about six drops of essential oil in an egg-cupful of dispersing oil. If this is not available, you can use vodka or full-cream milk as a base. Hot towels can be used as a compress with the added benefit of essential oils if you choose. Disperse a few drops of oil over the surface of a bowl containing very hot or ice cold water. Use a soft cloth to collect the oil from the surface, lightly squeeze out excess moisture and place the cloth over the affected area (probably your abdomen or lower back). A hot water bottle can also be very comforting on an aching back.

It's very important to remain hydrated during labour, as dehydration will increase distress. If you aren't at home, or your birthing environment doesn't provide purified water, make sure you have access to a plentiful supply, which is free of unhelpful toxins. You'll need to drink a lot, although hot drinks, such as non-herbal teas and coffee that are very dehydrating, should be avoided.

HERBS

Herbs have been used to cope with stress and pain during childbirth (and pregnancy) since time immemorial. Herbal remedies can be taken as a tea (or infusion), or you can ask a herbalist to make up a mix of fluid extracts and advise you on dosage (this will vary according to the preparation). You will also find many herbal medicines in tablet or capsule form in health food shops, and these should have clear directions (and cautions for pregnancy) on the label. While staff in these shops may be able to advise you, we strongly recommend that you check all herbal preparations, whatever form they may take, with a qualified herbalist, or against our recommendations, regarding their safety (bearing in mind the stage of your pregnancy). Herbal teas are generally less potent than fluid extracts or tablets, and you're unlikely to overdose. Indeed, you may need to increase the frequency with which you drink them during acute situations, such as labour, to one cup every hour or so. Alternatively, you could use one of the more active forms of the herb.

How to make a herbal tea or infusion

1. For every 30 g (two tablespoons) of herb, pour on 600 mL of boiling water.
2. Let it steep (infuse) for at least 15 minutes to get the full benefit of the active ingredients.
3. Strain.
4. Drink a cupful three times daily (during late pregnancy).
5. Make a fresh brew every day, use it within 24 hours, or refrigerate.

For stress relief, herbal nervines (calming herbal remedies) can be wonderfully soothing. During labour you can choose from (or mix together) *Chamomile* and *Lavender Flowers*, *Lemon Balm*, *Catnip*, *Green Oats*, *Zizyphus*, *Valerian*, *Linden*, *Vervain*, *Skullcap*, *Basil* and *Rosemary*. *Motherwort* is not only an excellent nervine and reproductive system tonic, but also helpful for palpitations (though it should not be used before week 36 of your pregnancy, as it can stimulate your uterus). *Hawthorn* may also be helpful for palpitations, but, again, supervision is required. *Cramp Bark* is not only calming, but helpful for the pain of contractions. *Withania* is a wonderful tonic for any stress in pregnancy and can help to boost your energy levels, as can *Damiana* (an anti-depressant). All of these can be used during labour, but some are better avoided during pregnancy, when the safest herbs to use are *Lemon Balm*, *Catnip*, *Withania*, *Green Oats* and *Zizyphus*. *Chamomile* can be extremely calming, but it is preferable to use only small doses and not for extended periods of time (two cups of tea a day should be fine). You'll soon discover your preferred herb or combination.

Herbs for pain relief

As far as pain relief goes, herbs work best as relaxants and preparators. A partus preparator or birth preparation tonic, taken during the last few weeks of pregnancy, will help to achieve the following:

- Improved uterine and cervical 'tone'.
- A labour that starts on time.
- Short labour.
- Rhythmic, regular and effective contractions.
- Minimal bleeding.
- A uterus that returns quickly to pre-pregnancy size.

- Plentiful supply of nutritious breast milk.
- Quick recovery/no exhaustion after the birth.

You can take these preventative, tonic herbs even if you're feeling fine, and they'll also help to ensure that those last few weeks are trouble-free, at a time when problems can escalate and threaten to complicate the birth. (Good daily nutritional support through both your diet and supplementation also constitute an important tonic at this time.)

Partus preparator herbs tone the uterine muscles, gently relax and reduce pain and tension in labour. *Parturient* herbs help the entire process of giving birth and assist in the smooth delivery of the placenta. The nervine herbs we've already discussed are also invaluable in this preparatory role, especially *Withania*, a traditional pregnancy tonic held in high esteem by practitioners of Ayurvedic medicine in India. Here's a list of herbs which could be helpful at this time.

- *False Unicorn Root* is a uterine tonic, hormone balancer and partus preparator herb.

- *Squaw Vine* is a uterine tonic, parturient, partus preparator and tonic for the urinary tract and bowels. It has also been used traditionally to support lactation and prevent bleeding.

- *Raspberry Leaf* is a parturient, haemostatic (controls bleeding), and reproductive tonic specific to pregnancy and childbirth. Some questions have been raised about its use in early pregnancy, and suggestions made that traditionally the wild raspberry (*Rubus strigosus*) was harvested and used (giving rise to the herb's reputation), whereas today most preparations are made from *Rubus idaeus*. Raspberry is high in calcium and magnesium, which help to strengthen and calm uterine muscles.

- *Nettle* is a wonderful tonic for the entire pregnancy. It supports the uterus, kidneys and urinary tract, increases available haemoglobin, strengthens blood vessels, helps maintain arterial elasticity and improves venous resistance. It protects against diabetes, poor digestion, fluid retention, incontinence, anaemia, hypertension, kidney stones, hair loss, leg cramps, painful childbirth, hypoglycaemia and a slow metabolic rate. These effects are partly due to *Nettle*'s high content of nutrients such as calcium, magnesium, iron, silica, copper, phosphorus, vitamins A, C, D and K, and chlorophyll. It will even increase the quality and quantity of your breast milk—you can see why we include it here! You can drink large amounts quite safely—up to a litre daily if you can manage it.

Wild Yam is a hormonal regulating, anti-inflammatory and antispasmodic herb which can reduce irritable cramping and stress and is a good liver tonic. It can also help prevent premature labour, and is very safe to take during both pregnancy and labour.

Cramp Bark and *Black Haw* are two herbs from the same family and have similar properties—they calm and relieve anxiety, prevent irregular and spasmodic uterine contractions, and help to reduce arterial blood pressure. They are also parturients, reduce the risk of premature labour and tonify the urinary tract. Both herbs are safe to take in pregnancy and during labour.

Dong Quai is used traditionally as a partus preparator in Chinese medicine. It brings a good supply of blood to the uterus and helps to correct cardiac arrhythmias and anaemia. (It should not be used in the first trimester of pregnancy, especially if you have a tendency to spontaneous abortion, and some authorities recommend to use it only after week 34. It's also contraindicated if you are bleeding.)

Peony is a uterine and hormonal regulator, and is also an antispasmodic. It combines well with *Dong Quai*, and these two herbs are used as a traditional Chinese formula—they are effective for painful Braxton-Hicks contractions. *Peony* is called the 'foetal calmer'.

Mugwort is another traditional Chinese partus preparator. (Do not use it before week 34 of your pregnancy.)

St Mary's Thistle is a bitter (which helps digestion), a galactagogue (which helps milk production) and an excellent herb for the liver (keeps all those hormones and toxins under control).

Beth Root is anti-haemorrhagic (prevents excessive bleeding) and a parturient. It's also known as 'Birth Root' because of its traditional use.

- *Black Cohosh* is an anti-spasmodic and sedative herb, which relaxes the cervix and uterine muscles, and regulates blood supply to the womb. However, its use and dosage should be professionally supervised.

- *Blue Cohosh* is a partus preparator and uterine tonic that has been traditionally and extensively used to facilitate labour and delivery. However, the dosage and use of this herb must be professionally supervised, or it may lead to excessive contractions and can adversely affect the foetus. If, while taking this herb, you notice any marked change in your baby's behaviour, you should discontinue use, though this is very unlikely if you use the herb correctly. Possible side-effects for the mother include headaches, dizziness and nausea. Despite these potential problems, it is a very helpful and widely used herb, both before and during childbirth (though it should only be taken for the last three weeks of pregnancy, because of its ability to initiate contractions). It's best to be cautious and begin with small doses, and then increase these as your due date approaches (or passes). Ask your herbalist for the correct dosage of the preparation you are using.

- *Withania* is a traditional pregnancy tonic herb used for centuries in India which is helpful to relieve stress, help sleep and boost flagging energy.

A possible partus preparator formula would be:

False Unicorn Root	20 mL
Squaw Vine	30 mL
Red Raspberry Leaf	45 mL
St Mary's Thistle	35 mL
Nettle	20 mL
Withania	50 mL
	200 mL

These dosages are based on the use of a 1:2 fluid extract.

As a preventative, this mix (or an equivalent) could be started at the thirty-fourth week of pregnancy, building the dose as follows:

Week 34: 2 mL per day	Week 37: 5 mL twice daily
Week 35: 2 mL twice daily	Week 38: 5 mL three times daily
Week 36: 2 mL three times daily	Week 39: 8 mL three times daily

If Braxton-Hicks contractions become too strong, you should stop the mix and start again, after a few days, on a lower dose, adding some anti-spasmodic herbs like *Cramp Bark*, *Black Haw* and *Wild Yam* to the formula. If you don't have access to fluid extracts, drinking *Raspberry* and *Squaw Vine* teas during the last few weeks of pregnancy will be helpful.

FLOWER ESSENCES

Flower essences can safely be used during the weeks leading up to the birth of your baby and also during labour to help you overcome stress. These are prepared in homoeopathic dosage (see below), and a few drops will be sufficient, though it's safe to take them as frequently as you feel the need. These essences may be particularly helpful at this time.

* *Aspen* for those vague, unformed fears which have no real target.

* *Beech* in case you're starting to snap at your nears-and-dears.

* *Cerato* for those who feel inadequate and keep seeking confirmation from others.

* *Cherry Plum* for when you feel a panic attack coming on.

* *Clematis* for lack of interest in the present; inattentiveness.

* *Elm* for those overwhelmed by responsibility: too much other stuff going on when you want to focus on your belly and your baby.

* *Gentian* for discouragement.

* *Hornbeam* for weakness, doubting the strength to cope.

* *Impatiens* in case it all suddenly seems to be taking too long, or you're getting irritable.

* *Larch* for lack of confidence that all will be well.

* *Mimulus* for those fears and anxieties about known problems.

* *Olive* for complete exhaustion.

❋ *Rock Rose* in case you are frightening yourself with images of disaster.

❋ *Vervain* for tension or hyper-anxiety.

❋ *Walnut* for protection from change and outside influences; in case people are telling you horror stories.

❋ *White Chestnut* for those worrying thoughts that won't go away, but play on like a record stuck in a groove (especially when you should be sleeping).

These are all remedies from the Bach Flower range, developed in England in the 1930s by Dr Edward Bach. Many countries have developed their own native flower essence ranges, which some feel relate better to contemporary concerns. The Australian Bush Flower range, developed by Ian White, has the following useful remedies for late pregnancy and childbirth.

❋ *Billy Goat Plum* to accept changing body shape.

❋ *Five Corners* as for Billy Goat Plum.

❋ *Dog Rose* for fear of labour and a sense of insecurity.

❋ *Fringe Violet* to protect against the negative influence of other people's experience.

❋ *Grey Spider Flower* for terror about the coming birth process, to encourage calm, courage and faith.

❋ *Illawarra Flame Tree* for feeling overwhelmed by responsibility.

A particular favourite for most labouring mums is *Rescue Remedy*, a combination of several Bach Flower remedies which is specific for times of crisis or exceptional demand.

HOMOEOPATHIC REMEDIES

Homoeopathy works by introducing minute amounts of herbal or mineral substances to the body, which trigger a response of self-healing, either in the body or in the mind. As the amounts used are infinitesimally small (and may not even be traceable on analysis) they have no potential for toxicity and are therefore an excellent choice for the pregnant or birthing mother, especially as their effect can be powerful and immediate.

The use of homoeopathy to control stress and pain before and during birth has been the subject of several studies in the UK. In one of these studies, a remedy of *Arnica, Caulophyllum, Cimicifuga, Pulsatilla* and *Gelsemium* was given for one month before birth in a double-blind, placebo-controlled study. This resulted in an average birth time that was almost four hours shorter than that of the control group, with a substantially lower rate of difficult births (11 per cent against 40 per cent).

If you want to use homoeopathic remedies to best advantage during this special time of late pregnancy and childbirth, it would be beneficial to consult with a homoeopath during the last trimester, so that an individualised homoeopathic kit could be prepared for you. We make some suggestions below and your support people could familiarise themselves with the use of each remedy. Where a symptom (such as thirst) is given as an 'indication' for a remedy, this does not necessarily mean that the remedy is being given to alleviate that particular symptom, but that the symptom indicates that this is the appropriate remedy to use. Remedies come in various potencies, but either '30c' or '6c' should be appropriate. We're grateful to Vicki Turner, a homoeopath who works at the Jocelyn Centre with Francesca, for suggesting the following remedies:

- *Aconite:* for fear and anxiety about birth and labour, restlessness, sudden sinking of strength, intolerable pain with anxiety and pains that are sharp, violent and rapid, and to allay shock. This remedy is also indicated if you have a desire for cold drinks.

- *Arnica:* this remedy can be taken at the '30c' potency once a day for approximately three days prior to your expected due date, and is more effective if the pilule is crushed into a powder. The dose should be repeated at the start of labour, and again just before delivery. This remedy can help to make labour faster and less painful as it helps muscle relaxation. It also relieves bruising to tissue and muscles. It is indicated if you feel like responding with, 'Don't touch me, I'm okay', when offered help during labour; if you are intolerant of physical examination due to physical sensitivity; if you change position often; if you are quarrelsome and if you feel heat only in your head, with flushing in your face. You should take no more than six doses of the '30c' potency remedy, or 10 doses of the '6c' potency.

Belladonna: for bearing down pains; for back pain that feels as if your 'back will break', or for pain drawing from the small of the back down the thighs. This remedy is indicated if your face and head are hot, red and flushed and your pulse is bounding, or if you feel worse for any jarring, noise or light.

Carbo Vegetabilis: for total exhaustion during a long labour.

Caulophyllum: to soften the cervix during labour, or for short, irregular and spasmodic pains. This remedy is the homoeopathic version of the herb *Blue Cohosh* (*Caulophyllum* is the herb's botanical name). It has none of the potential problems of the herb as far as causing early labour is concerned, and can be started at the '30c' potency, from the 37th week and taken once a week (on the same day). It will encourage regular and well-spaced contractions, tone the uterus, facilitate delivery and prevent premature labour. This remedy is indicated if you experience fever and thirst, and it's also useful for painful Braxton-Hicks contractions in the last few weeks of pregnancy.

Chamomilla: for unbearable labour pains, intolerance of strong pain or of touch, or for erratic, spasmodic pains which start in your back and pass down to your inner thighs. This remedy is indicated if you are irritable, fretful, restless, easily distracted, have temper tantrums or desire fresh air and fluids.

China: for great debility, vertigo, fainting and ringing in the ears, or for irritability, over-active mind, intolerance to noise. This remedy is indicated if your face and body feel cold, you want to be fanned or gasp for breath.

Cimicifuga: for fear of labour and pain, gloom.

Cocculus: for spasmodic, irregular pains in the small of your back, or for feelings of exhaustion and lack of control.

Coffea: for contractions that are very painful but irregular; for agitation and restlessness.

✳ *Gelsemium:* to soften the cervix during labour; for extreme anxiety, trembling and nervousness *or* drowsiness, lassitude and muscular weakness; for dull, heavy pain. This remedy is indicated if anxiety is accompanied by diarrhoea, general shakiness and trembling, or if the pain goes into the back and hips. It's also good for painful Braxton-Hicks contractions.

✳ *Ipecacuanha:* for nausea, vomiting or desire to vomit. This remedy is indicated if you feel faint, have a weak pulse, are gasping for breath or breathing heavily, or your head is hot with a cold sweat.

✳ *Kali Carb:* for back pain, especially sharp cutting pains across your lumbar region and in your buttocks, and for weakness felt in the small of your back or a burning sensation in your spinal column. This remedy is indicated if you have difficulty moving about, if you feel the need for something firm pressed into your back, or your pains are improved by belching. It's also an excellent remedy for exhaustion, or if you feel indifferent, disconnected or depressed.

✳ *Millefolium:* can be taken as a preventative remedy, in the '30c' potency, if heavy bleeding was experienced in a previous pregnancy.

✳ *Nat Mur:* for feelings of indifference, disconnectedness or depression (you can also try *Kali Carb* or *Sepia*).

✳ *Nux Vomica:* for lumbar pains that extend to the thighs or the rectum; for great irritability or sensitivity to touch, light, noise or odour. This remedy is indicated if you have a constant desire to urinate or defecate, even if doing so does not relieve the desire.

✳ *Pulsatilla:* for emotional vulnerability, weepiness, worry, and for sacral pains or those which constantly change position and intensity. This remedy is indicated if you faint (or feel faint), crave company and sympathy, lack any thirst, crave fresh air, want to be warm, feel breathless or want to walk around the room for relief of pain. It can also be given, in the '200c' potency, as a constitutional remedy, if you fit this emotional stereotype.

⊰ *Sepia:* for feelings of depression, indifference or disconnectedness (you can also try *Nat Mur* or *Kali Carb*).

⊰ *Virburnum:* this is the homoeopathic version of *Cramp Bark,* an antispasmodic and nervine, good for painful Braxton-Hicks contractions.

STRESS-BEATING NUTRIENTS

If you've regularly taken calcium and magnesium supplements (in a 2:1 ratio) during your pregnancy (see Chapter 4), you will have improved uterine muscle tone and your nervous system will be in better shape to cope with the stresses of childbirth. (Nettle tea is also an excellent source of these two important nutrients.) Both these minerals, which are nature's own sedatives, are in great demand during pregnancy, being used to form your baby's skeleton, and mums-to-be can easily become depleted, setting you up for a more stressful experience. If you are feeling irritable, anxious or nervous, or you are suffering from leg cramps or painful Braxton-Hicks contractions, you can take higher doses than usual (or start taking doses even if it's late in your pregnancy) and the most bio-available forms (most readily absorbed) are the tissue salts, calcium phosphate and magnesium phosphate, which can be safely taken every few hours. You may find these in your health food store in a form that dissolves under your tongue, which is ideal for use during childbirth (or for painful Braxton-Hicks contractions).

The B-complex vitamins are also reduced by stress, and you may need to temporarily increase your dosage as birth approaches. The same goes for vitamin C.

Good nutritional status can also help keep your energy levels high and avoid fluctuating blood sugar levels which can cause extreme fatigue and lead to stress. To stabilise blood sugar levels, keep snacking, eating little and often, especially light proteins such as nuts (almonds are particularly helpful), whole grains and seeds. Keep away from the sugar bowl! If you eat sugary snacks or too many high-glycaemic foods, any temporary increase in energy is likely to be followed by a crash. If you have kept your chromium levels stable during pregnancy, through supplementation, this is less likely to be a problem, though it's never too late to start. (Try double the maximum dose suggested in Chapter 4 if it's just a short-term, last-ditch effort.)

Blood sugar levels are a major concern during labour, and though some childbirth guides suggest taking sugary food and fruit juices into the birthing room, these are likely to cause as many problems as they solve. Even unsweetened fruit juices are very high in fructose and should be seen as a 'sugar hit'. If you really want them, dilute them half-and-half with purified water, and use sparingly.

SLEEP AND REST TO COMBAT STRESS

We've mentioned the importance of getting enough sleep in late pregnancy, both to help you get through the last few weeks and also so that you are well rested if labour starts in the middle of the night. However, there's no need to feel that as soon as labour begins there will be no more chance to sleep—early labour can be quite protracted, and though sleep may be disturbed by contractions, you may still be able to snatch a few more hours. The herbal nervines and acupressure points suggested earlier in this chapter will help you relax enough to be able to sleep. If you can't, or if early labour occurs during the day, it's still really important to relax as fully as possible between contractions, especially for a first labour which can take longer than those for subsequent births.

Although we can't promise you a pain-free birth experience, or even one that's completely lacking in stress, we do firmly believe that the measures we've outlined here can make a real and significant difference. Although any birth which brings a healthy child into the world can be considered a 'good birth', we'd like to think that this very special time can be even 'better'.

Your birth plan ... and beyond

Once you've chosen where, how and with whom you want to give birth to your baby, you should sit down with your partner and carefully work out your birth plan. When you both feel absolutely comfortable with this plan, you should discuss it with your carer and your other attendants. You must be satisfied that everybody who is supporting you and caring for you understands your wishes and will make every effort to see that your plan is implemented.

We've listed below some ideas you might want to incorporate in your plan. We're not suggesting that these requests are like the ten commandments. You may agree with some of them, but feel uncomfortable with others. However, if you're really keen to have a better birth and better bonding, they'll give you a starting point from which to work. You can incorporate whatever else is right for you and omit whatever doesn't fit in with your wishes and your particular situation.

A SAMPLE BIRTH PLAN

- I do not want to be induced

- I want non-invasive tests (such as cardiotocograph) for placental function if my baby is overdue

- I want to keep a 'kick chart' to record my baby's movements if I'm overdue

- I will alert my midwife as soon as I'm sure I'm in labour

- I will alert my support people as soon as I'm in real labour

- I want to go to the hospital/birth centre as late as possible

- I want to keep active in the early stages of labour (if I'm awake)

- I want to try to get some rest (if labour starts during the night)

- I don't want an enema/suppository to empty my bowels

- I don't want regular internal examinations

- I don't want my membranes ruptured to stimulate my labour

- I don't want syntocinon or prostaglandin gels to stimulate labour

- I want dim lights and a very warm room

- I want cushions/bean bags/oil burner/music

- I want to be free to move around at all times

- I want to be able to use the shower/bath/birth pool at any time

- I want to be able to deliver in the water if it feels right

- I want to be reminded to empty my bladder at regular intervals

- I want to be free to eat or drink if I want to

- I want to be free to use massage, acupressure, aromatherapy oils, hot packs, cold packs or whatever else might be appropriate for pain relief

- I don't want a time limit on first stage

- I want my partner to stay with me whatever happens

- I want my support people with me at all times

- I want my children with me, but only if they're comfortable

- I do not want to be offered gas for pain relief

- I do not want electronic foetal monitoring (EFM)

- I do not want to be offered an epidural

- I do not want an episiotomy

- I do not want a forceps delivery

- I want to be allowed to deliver in whichever position feels most comfortable

- I want my partner to assist with the birthing of our baby

- I want to hold my baby as soon as he is born

- I want to breastfeed as soon as my baby is ready to nurse

- I do not want weighing/measuring/washing straight after the birth

- I want the room warm enough so that I can have skin to skin contact with my baby

- I don't want my baby to be wrapped

- I want the umbilical cord to stop pulsing before it is cut

- I want the delivery of the placenta to proceed spontaneously

- I want to save the placenta (please freeze it for me)

- I want no interruptions to bonding

- I want to go home as soon as my baby is born

- I want my baby to room in; I do not want him to be taken to the nursery

- I want to have my baby in bed with me

- I want to feed my baby on demand

- I do not want my baby to have anything other than colostrum and breast milk

⚘ I want to delay bathing my baby until I get home

⚘ I don't want my baby to have Vitamin K injection/oral dose

⚘ I want to hold my baby while he has the Newborn Screening test

⚘ I want to be involved in any decisions that are going to affect me or my baby

⚘ I nominate . . . . to make these decisions on my behalf if I no longer feel able to do so myself

⚘ If I have any intervention such as an epidural, I want my partner to be present

⚘ If I have a Caesarean, I want my partner present and I want him to hold the baby immediately afterwards.

Chances are if you present this list to some obstetricians they'll politely tell you that such a plan is impossible. But all of these wishes are valid and they're also achievable with some effort on your part and the co-operation and support of the right birth attendants. So if you get a completely negative response, find someone else who'll at least discuss the issues which might be of concern to them and see if you can agree on a compromise plan with which you can both live happily.

Above all, stay flexible yourself. There's a little saying that we both like, and which should probably be our theme song:

Q: 'How do you make God laugh?'

A: 'Tell him your plans!'

But seriously, make your birth plan and make it carefully. But be ready to let it go if it becomes necessary to do so, and don't beat yourself up if things didn't turn out quite the way you hoped.

WHAT YOU'LL NEED AT THE BIRTH

No matter where you plan to give birth—at home, in a birth centre or in hospital—most of the items you need are pretty much the same. We've included a general list here, but you'll also be given a specific list for the place you've chosen, and midwives and childbirth educators will also have their own ideas. You'll probably also have some ideas of your own.

For you

- 3 nightgowns (or long shirts) which open right down the front
- dressing gown or track suit (air conditioning can get chilly)
- warm socks (ditto, and besides, you can always walk around in them)
- slippers or flip-flops (hospitals frown on bare feet)
- 4 nursing bras (these quickly become saturated with milk in the early days after the birth)
- 12 terry towelling nursing pads
- 2 boxes of disposable nursing pads
- 3 packets of sanitary towels (maternity or super strength—stick on variety is best)
- 10 pairs of well fitting briefs
- tracksuit or loose shorts and T-shirt to wear home
- Walkman and tapes/CDs
- card games/Scrabble
- books/magazines
- camera/film
- aromatherapy oils and burner
- massage oil
- hot/cold pack
- small sponge to suck
- bean bag (the hospital or birthing centre may provide one)
- lip salve
- purified water
- herbal teas
- homoeopathic or herbal remedies for stress and for the birth
- wholefood (not sugary) snacks/drinks (for you and your support people)
- swimsuit for your support person (when he or she joins you in the birthing pool)
- hand mirror (to watch your baby's head crowning)
- 2 wash cloths
- your normal toilet kit
- tissues/soft toilet paper

- ear plugs
- writing paper/thank you cards
- your address book
- diary/pen
- coins/phonecard for the public phone

For your baby

If you're having your baby in hospital, he will probably wear hospital clothes and use their nappies. You can, if you wish, dress your baby in his own clothes and you'll certainly need to take his own clothes for the trip home. Otherwise you'll need the following.

- 36 terry towelling nappies
- 3 packets of nappy liners
- several packs of disposable nappies (newborn size). These are for emergencies only, as they are a major pollutant in the environment.
- nappy fasteners (get the type that aren't likely to jab your finger or your baby's delicate flesh)
- 4 pairs pilchers (the fluffy type)
- 6 terry towelling jump suits (size 00 or 0 rather than 000 which he'll outgrow very quickly)
- 4 singlets (the envelope-type neck is best)
- 2 cardigans
- 2 pairs bootees (if he's a winter baby)
- 2 hats
- 3 pairs socks
- 3 cotton blankets
- 1 shawl
- sling

Homebirth requirements

If you're having a homebirth, your midwife will bring her birth kit, but you'll need a big pot in which to sterilise her instruments when she arrives. Some weeks before the birth date, she'll also give you a list of what you'll need to provide. This will include a big plastic drop sheet for the floor or the bed.

Water birth requirements

If you're going to have a water birth at home, you'll need to hire a birthing pool. These are usually big enough so that your midwife and your partner can get in the pool with you. They also have padding around the edges so that it's comfortable for you to hang over the side. If you're planning to give birth at home in your bath or spa, make sure that you prepare some makeshift padding to serve the same purpose. The area surrounding the bath or spa must be sufficiently roomy for your midwife to be present. You may also need room for your partner and other support people.

Don't forget that you'll need to hire the pool well in advance and have it in the house for several weeks around the time your baby's due. You should also be aware of how much water your pool will hold—the average one holds about 100 gallons (455 litres). A gallon (4.55 litres) of water weighs 4.5 kilos, so if you're planning to give birth in your upstairs bedroom, be sure that the floor will take the weight (about 450 kilos). You should also check that your domestic water tank has sufficient capacity to fill the pool with water. Most domestic tanks hold about 40–70 gallons (182–318.5 litres) of hot water and the water in the pool needs to be approximately blood temperature (36.7°C).

WHAT YOU'LL NEED AFTER THE BIRTH

For your baby

We don't believe in having too many baby accessories—they are simply rampant consumerism at its worst. But if there's something you feel you can't do without, you could look in the *Trading Post* or try the local papers for second-hand items. Usually friends with older children are happy to pass on used equipment, clothes and toys (and often the children as well if you ask nicely). Just remember that your baby will be happiest when he's carried close at all times, and when he sleeps with you. So for the moment forget about the fancy nursery with bassinet, cot and change table, and definitely leave the Rolls Royce pram on the showroom floor. Apart from baby clothes and nappies, you really need very little extra equipment. Here are our suggestions.

- sling
- baby capsule fitted in your car
- sheepskin
- small baby bath (some are moulded to give your baby's head support which makes bathing very easy)—although you can always use the kitchen sink
- face cloths
- soft bath towels (your old ones will be a bit hard on your baby's skin)
- baby wipes
- almond (or other nut) oil for baby massage
- *Witch Hazel* (or other herbal extracts, see Chapter 12) for the cord
- nappy buckets
- cradle (for those times when you can't be in bed with your baby)

For you

The best thing you can have ready at home is support from family and friends. If your partner can organise paternity leave, tell him to do it—and for as long as possible! This support doesn't mean that other family members have to be camping in the house with you—this could be more hindrance than help—although it depends a great deal on how you all get on. Someone who calls by, unasked, with a ready made meal, puts on a load of washing and hangs it out, takes the older children for the day or does some shopping for you is a real blessing. If you don't have that kind of support—which is likely if you've been a career woman until now—don't be afraid to ask for it! Now is the time to call in a few favours. If this is your first baby, in those early weeks you'll be flat out getting yourself showered and out of your PJs by dinnertime, so accept any offers of help graciously and if they're not forthcoming ask for help.

If you can't bear the thought of your mother-in-law in residence, take the time to prepare a few meals well ahead of the expected arrival of your baby. Stock the freezer and the pantry as if you were bunkering down to withstand nuclear fallout. Then make every effort to do as little as possible—although those early days, which seem just an endless succession of feeding, bathing, feeding and more feeding won't be exactly like a health farm holiday. But it's important that you focus on your baby as much as you can in the early weeks. This might mean turning visitors away (unless of course they're coming to help, or with gifts of food). You don't want to be entertaining and making endless cups of tea for callers. This time is for you and your baby to get to know one another!

Don't be too keen to go out and about with your new baby either. He'll benefit from a gradual adjustment to his new environment, and will be much easier to settle and feed if he is introduced slowly to other family members, friends, car journeys, the local shops and the wider world. Pretty soon you'll be doing all sorts of things with him and taking him all sorts of places, but in the early weeks, staying close to home allows you both the chance to get into some sort of a routine and adjust to your new life together. It also gives your body time to recover physically from the pregnancy. Sheila Kitzinger refers to this time as the fourth trimester of pregnancy. Akal Khalsa, who has assisted at the births of over 1000 babies (700 of those at home) and who has generously offered her thoughts on the content of this book, is strident in her support of this advice. If this period for recovery and establishment of breastfeeding and your relationship with your baby is not respected, you will struggle through the next two years.

Forget about the superwoman act and allow yourself to be nurtured. This time is special for both you and your baby. Everything and everyone else can wait. Respect the wisdom of older cultures. Put your feet up— it's going to be a while before you get the opportunity again.

Natural or medical management?

chapter 9

Sometimes, despite the most nutritious diet, rigorous attention to a healthy lifestyle, an unswerving belief in the normality of the birth process, and a total commitment to avoiding any medical intervention, things don't always go according to plan. Despite your diligent attention to everything we've recommended, your carefully laid plans may come unstuck. Though in many situations you may be able to use natural remedies to avoid medical intervention this may not always be possible, and you might find yourself facing a 'high-risk' birth. Before you get too worried about this, let's look first of all at what does—and does not—constitute a high-risk birth, and what you can do to ameliorate the situation using natural remedies. Then, if medical management is necessary, we'll take a look at what you might expect to encounter and how best to face it.

WHAT CONSTITUTES A 'HIGH-RISK' BIRTH?

There are really three categories of risk. There are those conditions where the risk is high enough to be life threatening and many of these may necessitate a Caesarean section and will definitely require medical management and hospitalisation. Then there are those risks which are real problems, but can be managed in a number of ways, and may well result in a successful delivery without medical intervention. These are usually managed in a hospital environment, though a birthing centre may be willing to admit you. Some of the conditions in this category are even considered a manageable risk by certain home-birth midwives. You would need to discuss these conditions with your prospective carers to see if they have experience of, and confidence in their ability to manage, any specific condition that may arise. Your birth plan may need to be adapted according to the abilities of your carers. The last category of risk is that of conditions that can generally be handled quite safely outside a medical environment, but are frequently deemed to require it. These may often be successfully managed at home if you wish, depending on the experience and confidence of the midwife.

Conditions definitely requiring medical management

Some of these conditions will only require medical intervention if they are present during delivery, when they should definitely be managed in a hospital environment, and may require a Caesarean section. Remember, even if you are faced with one of these conditions (especially if this is in the later stages of pregnancy, before labour commences) you may still be able to use natural therapies in tandem with medical management to give yourself and your baby the best possible chance of an active, natural birth. As we discuss each condition we'll look at what you can do to help you and your baby.

Placenta praevia

In this condition the placenta has attached low down in the uterus below the baby. The risk of the baby's passage being blocked is higher the lower the attachment. Vaginal delivery is possible if the placenta does not obscure, or come too close to, the entrance to the womb. Otherwise a Caesarean will need to be performed. Placenta praevia diagnosed early in pregnancy on the basis of ultrasound may not persist, and may result in undue anxiety and an unnecessary Caesarean. Repeat ultrasounds, though we don't usually advocate them, may be necessary in this situation, and can prevent unnecessary surgery. All bleeding in late pregnancy should be investigated by your carer.

High blood pressure/pre-eclampsia (toxaemia)

Hypertension (raised blood pressure) can take two forms during pregnancy. Chronic hypertension is a commonly experienced slight rise which occurs in pregnancy because of the extra demands on your metabolism, increased blood volume and stress on the kidneys. This should not harm you or your baby, but needs to be watched carefully.

Gestational hypertension, or a steady rise in blood pressure after week 25, may be due to poor nutrition, especially a lack of protein (vegetarians beware, and read Chapter 4), which is commonly thought to be the main cause of toxaemia (also called pre-eclampsia). It may also mean that your placenta or kidneys are not functioning as well as they should. This condition has also been linked to a high body burden of toxic metals such as copper or lead, and occurs when the levels of essential minerals, especially zinc, are low. Toxaemia is more common in first pregnancies, and may not be a problem in subsequent pregnancies.

If your blood pressure does rise, it's important to start treating it quickly so it doesn't progress to toxaemia. Toxaemia means, literally, poisoning of the blood, so it's very important to keep your kidneys healthy, especially since they also have a role in maintaining normal blood pressure.

Pre-eclampsia is initially diagnosed by a steep rise in blood pressure, uric acid in the blood, a low urine output, fluid retention (oedema) and sudden weight gain. Singly, these symptoms may not be a cause for serious concern, but together they indicate pre-eclampsia. They may be accompanied by a general itchiness, and progress to a situation where protein appears in the urine. At this point there is a high risk of premature labour because of placental insufficiency which causes the blood flow to the foetus to be severely reduced, leading to a lack of oxygen.

Further symptoms, such as severe headaches, visual disturbances, nausea, vomiting and abdominal pain, mean that there is a threat of the condition progressing to eclampsia, which is characterised by fits and even coma. At the appearance of this second level of symptoms, or if the threat to the child becomes too severe, induction or a Caesarean section will be performed.

If you are supplementing as directed, eating well (especially adequate, quality protein), your kidneys are well supported (*Nettle* tea or acupuncture work best for this), and especially if you have no personal or family history of hypertension, there's a very good chance that you won't experience these problems. If you do, however, here are some remedies for the early stages. (Once the condition has progressed beyond these first stages, more aggressive therapy and medical supervision are required.)

- First, rest and relax. (See Chapters 6 and 7 for hints on controlling stress.)

- Avoid stimulants like cola drinks, teas and spicy foods.

- Exercise (see Chapter 5). Yoga is particularly helpful, but aerobic exercise is also excellent if it has been a regular part of your routine throughout pregnancy.

- Allow yourself a healthy weight gain—certainly don't diet! But, on the other hand, make sure to avoid fatty and sugary foods.

- Eat both calcium and protein-rich foods, keep the ratio of protein to (complex) carbohydrates as we've suggested in Chapter 4, and *sparingly* add salt (sea, rock or Celtic) to taste. To make sure that your salt requirements are not due to a depraved sense of taste, administer the Zinc Taste Test regularly and supplement appropriately (see Chapter 4).

- Drink plenty of purified water (2–3 litres daily).

- Drink *Nettle*, *Dandelion* and *Lime Flowers* teas regularly. *Hops* can also be helpful but only in the last trimester.

- Make sure you're taking adequate levels of vitamin E (for circulation), EPA/DHA (fish oils), vitamin B6, magnesium, calcium, potassium and zinc. Women suffering from pre-eclampsia have been found to be low in glutathione, which is symptomatic of poor antioxidant status, so make sure you get plenty of vitamins C and E, betacarotene and zinc. N-acetylcysteine (a nutritional supplement) may be particularly helpful as it is a precursor of glutathione.

⚹ If you feel that you have neglected your sources of calcium, magnesium and potassium and need a quick boost, use the celloids (or tissue salts) calcium phosphate, magnesium phosphate and potassium chloride, which are the most easily assimilated forms of these minerals. Potassium-rich foods include bananas, dandelion leaves, chicory, mint and potato peel. It's important to keep your potassium–sodium ratio high, which is why you need to go easy on the salt (without restricting it altogether, if you feel a genuine need for it). Raw beetroot juice is also very helpful.

⚹ Essential fatty acids (*Evening Primrose, Flaxseed* or deep-sea fish oils) have been successfully used in the treatment of pre-eclampsia.

⚹ The amino acid L-arginine has been shown to be helpful (but don't use this if herpes is a problem). See page 169 for a list of arginine-rich foods.

⚹ Herbs can reduce your stress levels (see Chapter 7). Try *Lemon Balm, Cramp Bark* and *Green Oats*.

⚹ *Garlic* should be a regular part of your diet and supplement regimen. Onions, parsley and cucumber are excellent foods too. Cucumbers, especially the yellow, over-ripe variety, are extremely effective in reducing blood pressure. You'll need a whole cucumber each day, or half a cup of juice, which may be easier to consume. This will also relieve constipation and strengthen your kidneys.

⚹ *Hawthorn* herb is specifically recommended for the treatment of high blood pressure. However, its use in pregnancy should be supervised and, although there is no documented proof of problems, it should be avoided if possible in the first trimester, and used with caution in the second. *Motherwort* and *Black Cohosh* can also help, but as we've mentioned before, their use must also be supervised and *Motherwort* should not be used before week 36. *Zizyphus* is a helpful herb that is safe in pregnancy.

⚸ Aromatherapy with *Lavender* can help.

⚸ Some studies have shown that reflexology is effective in controlling blood pressure and treating toxaemia. Treat the reflex areas for the heart, the kidneys and adrenal glands, and the urinary system.

⚸ Acupuncture or acupressure can also lower high blood pressure. Try 'dispersing' or 'calming' (see below) these points:
Stomach 9: three finger widths from the middle of the larynx (Adam's apple). With the thumb and middle finger of either hand, trace the crease line under your chin until you feel the larynx. Then press in and slightly away from the larynx, until you feel a pulse on one side of it. This is the spot you need.
Bladder 15: on either side of the spine, between the fifth and sixth thoracic vertebrae, behind the nipple line.
Bladder 22: on either side of the spine between the first and second lumbar vertebrae.

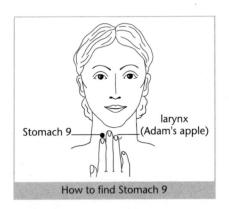

How to find Stomach 9

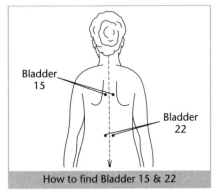

How to find Bladder 15 & 22

To disperse, apply moving pressure, such as a circular anti-clockwise motion, or a pumping action in and out on the point. The pressure can be begun fairly deep, then brought up to the surface. Take care to keep the area relaxed, and increase the pressure on successive treatments as your tolerance improves. To calm, cover the point with the palm of the hand or gently stroke for about two minutes.

Transverse lie

In this condition the baby is lying across the uterus. You may be able to correct this—see under 'Breech presentation' later in this chapter.

Pre-existing conditions

Pre-existing conditions such as cardiac disease, kidney disease, diabetes mellitus and epilepsy require medical management. You may be able to use natural therapies to treat these conditions prior to pregnancy or birth, though they will need professional supervision. Once you are in labour, medical management is necessary.

Herpes (if active in the vagina or vulva at the time of the birth)
Genital herpes may persist despite good preconception and pregnancy health care, as the virus is impossible to eradicate. It's a particular problem if there are lesions present in the birth canal at the time of delivery. An active infection can have severe repercussions for the baby, including brain damage, blindness and death, and a Caesarean section may be necessary. Even if the infection is dormant, an induction is sometimes recommended, to avoid an acute episode being triggered by labour. If the disease is first contracted during pregnancy (rather than recurrent attacks being experienced) there is an increased risk of miscarriage. However, natural remedies can be effective in keeping the virus dormant and in treating the blisters. The secret is to keep your immune system strong. The following may help.

- Eat well, as we have recommended, with an emphasis on fish, but avoid foods high in L-arginine (see box, page 169).

- No smoking, alcohol, drugs (of course!) or chocolate.

- Keep your dosages of zinc, manganese, magnesium, vitamins A (or preferably beta or mixed carotenoids), B1, B6 (with B-complex), E and C (with bioflavonoids) at recommended levels (as a minimum).

- Take the amino acid L-lysine (at 250 mg daily from four months of pregnancy, as a preventative, and 1000 mg daily for a week if an attack threatens) and avoid L-arginine. (See box, page 169, for lysine-rich foods.)

- Take *Evening Primrose* and deep-sea fish oils (or *Flaxseed* oils) and include raw seeds, fish and cold-pressed vegetable oils in your diet.

ℵ Take *Siberian Ginseng, Burdock, Calendula* and *St John's Wort* (these herbs in small doses only, and under supervision), *Echinacea, Lemon Balm, Cleavers, Reiishi* and *Shiitake* mushrooms, and *Garlic* to boost your immune response.

ℵ Keep your stress levels under control and get plenty of sleep and rest (see Chapter 7).

Warning signs

The warning signs of herpes include:
- Genital pain, itching, tingling pain with urination, vaginal discharge, tenderness in the groin;
- Fever, headache, general aches and pains, depression;
- Small red spots around and on the genitalia;
- Lymph node swelling in the groin.

Natural treatments

Once the warning signs are noted, and even before the blisters come out, you can apply the following remedies. Areas of severe itching and soreness are likely to be the sites of future blisters. Avoid sexual inter-course (or use a condom) to prevent infection passing back and forth.

ℵ Take *Garlic* in high dosage as soon as warning signs are felt and repeat the dose every three to four hours.

ℵ Increase dosage of immune stimulant herbs (see earlier in this section).

ℵ Apply ice to the site (on for 10 minutes, off for five).

ℵ Use *Witch Hazel, Calendula, Golden Seal, Myrrh* or *Solanum nigrum* as an extract or ointment, or apply *Aloe Vera* (best taken fresh from the inside of a fleshy stem) directly to the area. These herbs can also be used in a sitz-bath.

ℵ Cotton wool balls soaked in ether can be applied to reduce the pain. (Warning: ether is highly flammable.)

ℵ Use L-lysine cream on the site.

Foods high in lysine	Foods high in arginine
(helpful for herpes)	(helpful for pre-eclampsia, unhelpful for herpes)
• Fresh fish (100 g ≜ 1000 mg lysine)	• Nuts (especially almonds)
• Black beans/soy/lentils (1 cup ≜ 2500 mg lysine)	• Peanuts (this is actually a legume, not a nut)
• Watercress (½ cup ≜ 100 mg lysine)	• Seeds
• Chicken (organic and free range)	• Wheat (also most grains/ cereals)
• Beef (organic and free range)	• Brown rice
• Eggs (organic and free range)	• Oats
• Milk/dairy (not too much of this if it's from a cow)	• Chickpeas
• Yoghurt (this should be fine, even from a cow)	• Eggplants
• Sprouts	• Capsicums
• Vegetables	• Tomatoes
• Papaya	• Mushrooms
• Apricots	• Sugar (as if you would!)
• Pears	• Chocolate (as above)
• Apples	• Cocoa
• Figs	• Carob
	• Coffee
	• Caffeine (including soft drinks)
	• Raisins

✳ Apply zinc sulphate solution directly to the vaginal area.

✳ Essential oils which can be applied directly (though diluted or in a cream) include *Rose, Lavender, Geranium, Lemon, Sandalwood* and *Bergamot. Tea Tree* and *Hypericum* (*St John's Wort*) can also be used in this way, and all these oils can be used in a bath, as can Epsom salts (soak for at least 30 minutes).

✳ The homoeopathic remedies which may help include: *Rhus tox* (if there is pain and general aching); *Arsenicum* (if there is intense burning); *Hepar sulph* (if the blisters are painful when touched) and *Nat mur* (if the blisters are filled with liquid and on the vaginal labia).

➢ Acupuncture may also be useful: see your acupuncturist for effective treatment.

If this is not the primary outbreak your baby may have built up immunity during the pregnancy and this may ameliorate the threat.

Rhesus factor

If you are Rhesus negative and Rhesus antibodies are present in your blood there may be damage to your baby. It is necessary in these cases for your baby to have a blood transfusion directly after birth, to prevent the ill-effects. There are no remedies for this condition.

Prolapsed cord

In this condition the cord can be compressed by the baby's head and cause foetal distress, and a Caesarean section is necessary. This is often caused when the amniotic sac is ruptured prematurely in an attempt to induce labour.

Multiple pregnancy (three or more babies)

As multiple babies may be very small and vulnerable, they may need to be placed in humidicribs or on life-support systems initially.

Very low birth weight or premature babies (less than 2.5 kg/5½ lbs or less than 37 weeks)

The five per cent of Australian babies who arrive early, before 37 weeks or who weigh less than 2.5 kg, are considered premature, and this will usually necessitate medical management. But, though low birth weight is associated with an increased risk of problems of all kinds, if you have been assiduous in your health care and nutrition before and during pregnancy, your baby will be a lot better equipped to survive. Of course, these preparatory measures will also mean that you are less likely to experience a premature delivery, as good health and nutritional status are major factors in its prevention, and will also make it less likely that you suffer from any of the other known causes discussed elsewhere in this chapter, which include

➢ *Pre-eclampsia:* see previous section for remedies.

➢ *Premature rupture of the membranes:* good nutrition is essential here.

⚭ *Ovarian cysts and fibroids:* these can be treated naturally, though preferably before conception, as some of the most effective remedies are contra-indicated in pregnancy.

⚭ *Multiple conceptions:* we've no great ideas on how to avoid these! However, avoiding IVF or related procedures and fertility drugs is an important factor—see our previous book *A Natural Way to Better Babies* for more on overcoming fertility problems naturally.

⚭ *Placental insufficiency:* if you've followed our advice on pregnancy health care, this is also less likely to occur.

⚭ *Incompetent cervix:* can be affected very positively through natural medicines and nutrients. Medical management is through a stitch inserted in the cervix, and then removed in the thirty-eighth week. Though there are some risks involved, and this will not always be recommended, it is more common when the mother has experienced previous premature births or late-term miscarriage.

The first sign that you are going into labour prematurely may be that your waters break, you experience some vaginal bleeding, or that contractions commence, and this is usually completely unexpected. Most women are unaware of any risk, though women carrying more than one baby, those who have any structural abnormality of the uterus, placenta praevia, high blood pressure, diabetes, liver or kidney disease or genito-urinary infections may already be aware that they are more likely to give birth prematurely.

Most of the other reasons are to do with lifestyle issues such as poor nutrition, smoking, drinking alcohol, taking drugs (medicinal or social), experiencing high levels of stress, or taking part in unduly heavy physical activity, which can all cause labour to start before your baby is ready. We're not talking about reasonable levels of exercise here—as long as you're not causing excess strain, your baby is no more likely to become dislodged than, say, your kidneys (see Chapter 5 for more on exercise at this time). If you know that you are in a high-risk category, then you may wish to reduce the level of exercise, and even avoid sexual activity and orgasm in the last months of pregnancy, and some highly at-risk mothers may even require bed rest.

The earliest signs of premature labour can be a watery or pink discharge, the passing of a thick, jelly-like plug of mucus, a trickle of amniotic fluid, lower back or pelvic pain or pressure, sometimes accompanied by diarrhoea or nausea. Prompt attention is important, as each day your baby remains in the womb can make a great deal of difference. Bed rest alone can be enough in 50 per cent of cases where the contractions are not accompanied by bleeding (unless some other condition is complicating the situation).

If you suspect that your membranes have ruptured (waters have broken), you may not be sure if you have lost control of your bladder. As urine smells like ammonia, and amniotic fluid smells sweet, a quick sniff should help you decide. Also, as the amniotic fluid replaces itself every three hours, it will continue to leak. If your baby's head is already engaged, you can help to stem the flow by remaining erect, as then the head will act like a cork in a bottle. At this stage, you are likely to begin labour within the next 24 hours, but there is a risk of infection if you should take longer. Avoid sexual intercourse, baths, tampons and wiping faecal matter forwards to the vulval area, which should be kept as clean as possible. Use sanitary pads to absorb the fluid if the flow's not too great (otherwise you may need to wrap yourself in bath towels), and get in touch with your midwife (or doctor).

How early can we save lives?
Babies are being saved at earlier stages of pregnancy these days. Infants born as early as 24 weeks can survive, though it's a stressful fight. By 26 weeks there is a 50 per cent chance of survival and a 75 per cent chance of the baby being healthy if it lives. Medical teams make supreme efforts to save these very small babies, and this, of course, is a matter of great concern (and joy when it's successful) to the parents. However, prevention must always have priority over emergency rescue, especially as, tragically, many very low birth weight babies go on to have quite severe illnesses and disabilities. As society's priority must be the conception and birth of healthy, happy children, we have to question whether the vast amounts of money spent saving these heart-wrenching babies, who may subsequently suffer from disabilities such as cerebral palsy, blindness, deafness, mental retardation, chronic lung disease, learning disabilities or attention deficit disorder might not be better spent providing natural, holistic health care to parents both before and during conception, to

reduce significantly not only the possibility of the premature births, but also the incidence of children with a physical or health problem.

Preventing premature labour

If you are at risk of premature labour and your membranes are intact, you can take steps to prevent it. Even if your waters have broken, if the leaking stops and the membranes heal, you could use some of the preventative treatments listed below, though you should always take the advice of your midwife or obstetrician. She will monitor your baby's progress and condition. If he is distressed, it is better for labour to proceed so that he can receive appropriate care.

꙳ First, bed rest and relaxation.

꙳ Avoid lifting heavy objects and always bend your knees (not your back) with any lifting.

꙳ A warm bath can be very relaxing (going to the bathroom should be the only time you get out of bed), and you could use some of the relaxing, soothing essential oils we've recommended in Chapter 7. Bath water should be lukewarm, since heat can stimulate the uterus.

꙳ Warmth is nurturing to the uterine environment, so avoid cold drinks and food. Warm foods such as soups and casseroles, root vegetables and herbal teas are comforting as well as therapeutic.

꙳ On the other hand, don't get too hot! Heat, stress and dehydration can increase the risk of premature labour, so drink lots of purified water. Just make sure it's at room temperature, not iced or straight from the fridge.

꙳ Avoid intercourse, or any sexual stimulation, since this may 'excite' the uterus. Penetration is definitely contraindicated if your membranes have ruptured.

꙳ Important nutrients at this time include magnesium and vitamins C and E. Magnesium can be taken as the tissue salt magnesium phosphate, to prevent cramping. It can be combined with calcium phosphate, and taken at least three to four times daily. This can safely be taken in addition to your daily dose of magnesium (see Chapter 4). Vitamin C and the bioflavonoids are important for capillary integrity, and can reduce any bleeding (see Chapter 4 for recommended dosages). Vitamin E may help to strengthen the attachment of the placenta, and thereby reduce the chance of miscarriage. However, do not exceed the recommended dose (see Chapter 7), since too much may cause overly-strong attachment. This could lead to a problem in the third stage of labour when the placenta is expelled. Also, if your blood pressure is elevated, get advice from your health practitioner regarding dosage.

- 'Rescue Remedy' is the appropriate flower essence at this time.

- Visualise your baby being held in your womb by a 'safety net' of white light that calms your uterus and protects him. Talk to your baby and ask him to stay in your belly until the time is right for his entrance into the world (which may, just possibly, be now). Surround him with your love.

- Reflexology may be helpful. Try massaging the areas of the solar plexus (to calm and relax you), and the pelvic area (see the diagram in Appendix 1). This should only be attempted if premature labour threatens after 34 weeks' gestation.

- Herbs that are useful at this time include the anti-spasmodics *Cramp Bark*, *Black Haw*, *Wild Yam* and *Peony*. Uterine tonics such as *False Unicorn Root* and *Dong Quai* may also help (though don't use *Dong Quai* if you're bleeding), as can *Raspberry* and *Squaw Vine*, which may also act to prevent bleeding. *Valerian* and *Chamomile* can help to calm both your emotions and your womb.

- Medical management of premature labour may include the use of drugs to delay contractions for up to 48 hours. However there is no evidence that these actually reduce rates of perinatal mortality or improve birth weight. Cortisone drugs may also be used for babies who are born before 36 weeks to speed up the maturation of their lungs.

Foetal distress (depending on progress of labour)
If your baby's heartbeat shows that he is in distress, intervention may be necessary, unless the delivery is imminent. Of course much of this distress may be the direct result of interventions.

Bright red bleeding during first stage of labour

This indicates possible placenta praevia or abruptio placenta (when the placenta separates from the womb). Though medical supervision is necessary, *Raspberry*, *Squaw Vine* and *Nettle* are mild haemostatic (anti-haemorrhagic) herbs, and *Shepherd's Purse* and *Beth Root* have a stronger action. You'll find more herbs and homoeopathic remedies for blood loss below. If the bleeding is during late pregnancy, an ultrasound will need to be performed to ascertain the position of the placenta, and there are some preventative remedies that you can use. Vitamin E has been shown to improve placental attachment, and may be useful. The appropriate dosage is 500–800 IU daily (see Chapter 4) or 1000 IU for a short time only (for the duration of the problem). Vitamin C and the bioflavonoids are important for capillary integrity, and may help if the bleeding is from the cervix. The homoeopathic remedy *Millefolium* can also be taken, in the '30c' potency, as a preventative.

Haemorrhage

It's quite natural to have some bleeding after the birth of your baby, and you will probably experience three to four days of red discharge (called lochia) which fades to brownish-pink and then to white or clear by about the ninth day. It can sometimes take as long as six weeks to stop altogether. If you continue to have bright red bleeding or clotting, there may be some retained placental tissue, and you should talk to your midwife or doctor. You may find massage of the reflex zone for the uterus helps (see diagrams page 279). If you have a fever, or a bad smelling discharge, there may be infection, in which case *Echinacea* herb, vitamin C and *Garlic* can be used. You may need a course of antibiotics as well. If this is the case, make sure to supplement with *Acidophilus* and *Bifidus* to keep your intestinal flora intact. These helpful bacteria which live in your gut are essential for producing vitamin K, which assists blood clotting.

There are several possible causes of excessive blood loss, including the failure of your uterus to contract back to its original size (involution). For this you can use any of the remedies we've suggested for inefficient contractions. Retention of the placenta (see below), an injury in the cervix or uterus (for example if forceps have been used), or a clotting disorder (see our recommendations in Chapter 10 for sources of vitamin K) are other reasons for abnormal bleeding.

If the bleeding persists, and you lose more than 500 mL within

24 hours of delivery, either through sudden gushes with large clots, or through a constant, though moderate, flow, then you are haemorrhaging. Medical intervention is necessary, as this blood loss can have very serious effects and may require drug injections or even a blood transfusion. The risk of haemorrhaging is greater if this is your fourth or subsequent baby, if you had a long labour, or if your haemoglobin levels are low. If you've been drinking *Nettle* tea, and following our recommendations for avoiding anaemia (see page 186), your risk will be much reduced.

If you are bleeding, it may be preferable to use herbs as an infusion, since fluid extracts and tinctures contain alcohol which can stimulate circulation and increase the blood loss. Alternatively, you can use tablets or powders, and you may need small, frequent doses. Professional supervision is always necessary, as the condition can deteriorate very rapidly. The traditional Chinese herb for postpartum bleeding is *Tienchi Ginseng* (not for use in pregnancy), and other herbs include:

- Astringent herbs such as *Beth Root, Periwinkle, Motherwort, Raspberry, Ladies Mantle, Witch Hazel, Yarrow, Golden Seal* and *Shepherd's Purse;*

- Oxytocic herbs (those that encourage the release of oxytocin, which helps your uterus to contract) such as *Blue Cohosh* and *Golden Seal;*

- Herbs containing vitamin K such as *Nettle, Alfalfa* and *Shepherd's Purse.*

There's also a wide range of homoeopathic remedies to choose from. Remember that these have no potential for toxicity and the effects can be powerful and immediate. Ideally, you'll have the help of a professional homoeopath, or your midwife or support person will have familiarised themselves with the full list of remedies (which you should keep available). The dose, in this acute situation, should be of the '200c' potency.

- *Aconite:* for bleeding with fear of death.

- *Arnica:* if bleeding is due to injury.

- *Belladonna:* if bleeding is profuse, hot and bright red, and your face and head are also hot and red, and your pulse is bounding.

- *Carbo vegetabilis:* for haemorrhage with imminent collapse; if you are very pale, cold, with a cold sweat, and want fresh air.

- *Caulophyllum:* for bleeding after an exhausting, hasty or swift labour, and if you are trembling and weak.

- *China:* for profuse bleeding with exhaustion, great debility or fainting, loss of sight or ringing in the ears.

- *Hamamelis:* if, despite a slow and steady loss of blood, you are not concerned or anxious.

- *Ipecachuana:* for sudden gushes of bright red blood, and if you are gasping for breath and nauseated, with a hot head but cold sweat.

- *Phosphorus:* for persistent, bright bleeding which stops and starts, with feelings of weakness, cold, emptiness in the abdomen, and if your back feels 'broken' and hot.

- *Sabina:* for dark blood with severe uterine pain.

Retention of the placenta

If the placenta does not come away cleanly it can cause haemorrhage or infection. However, given sufficient time, and immediate breast-feeding, the third stage of labour usually results in its easy expulsion. If it doesn't come away easily and cleanly, your midwife or obstetrician may attempt to remove it manually. You can help by assuming a squat-ting position, and pushing, as you did during the second stage of labour. It will also help if your baby is at your breast and suckling, if you stimulate your nipples and gently massage your uterus.

Calcium and magnesium, in tissue salt form, will help your uterus to contract and expel the placenta, as will the herbs we've suggested before, such as *Raspberry, Golden Seal, Dong Quai, Blue* and *Black Cohosh, Beth Root, Mugwort, Ginger* and *Feverfew. Basil* and *Catnip* can also help. The homoeopathic remedies include *Arsenicum, Bella-donna* and *Caulophyllum* (see the last section for special indications). You may also find these additional remedies helpful:

- *Arsenicum:* if you are restless but exhausted, and are short of breath on exertion.

- *Cantharsis:* if there are burning pains in the ovaries or 'os' (the cervical opening), with urination which is painful (though it helps to expel the placenta) or constant discharge.

- *Gelsemium:* if your contractions are ineffectual.

- *Pulsatilla:* if your contractions are slow and you feel emotionally vulnerable.

- *Sepia:* if there are bearing down pains in the uterus.

Conditions which may require medical management

Prolonged rupture of membranes
If this is not followed by the commencement of labour within 24 hours, there will be a risk of infection, and your doctor may recommend induction. However, as the amniotic fluid constantly renews itself, observation may be sufficient.

Premature rupture of membranes
Hospitalisation is necessary if your membranes rupture before 37 weeks, so the baby's progress can be monitored, and your temperature watched for signs of fever, indicating infection, which will require medication and induction.

Treatment in this situation will vary according to whether labour (spontaneous or induced) ensues. A small rupture, resulting in a continuous but moderate loss of fluid, may heal spontaneously. The risk of infection may be the deciding factor in the decision to induce and this is usually carried out within 12–24 hours. However, one study showed that this risk only increased significantly after four days. Another risk factor to consider is the degree of prematurity. If your midwife or obstetrician suggests that it's worth waiting, there are several measures you can take to assist the healing process.

- Vitamins C and E, betacarotene and zinc are important nutrients for the integrity of the membranes. Hopefully you've been taking these all through your pregnancy as a preventative measure. If not, start now! (See Chapter 4 for dosages.) Vitamin C will also help to protect against infection, as will the herbs *Echinacea* and

Calendula (in small doses and with professional supervision), and *Garlic*.

⚜ Continue with the herbal teas we suggested as a birth preparation 'tonic'—*Raspberry*, *Squaw Vine* and *Nettle*—and if there is any bleeding add *Shepherd's Purse* and *Beth Root*. You can ask your herbalist to supply these in the form of fluid extracts for greater effectiveness. The anti-spasmodic herbs *Cramp Bark*, *Black Haw*, *Wild Yam* and *Peony* will help to prevent contractions.

⚜ Lie down *immediately* and move as little as possible for at least 48 hours, or until the leaking stops.

⚜ Visualise protection for your child, seeing your membranes as intact, strong and healthy.

⚜ Make sure that there is no exposure to microbial infection—pay great attention to hygiene. When you have a bowel motion, wash the perineum and rectum with water. A good way to manage this is to use a 'peri-bottle', which you can improvise from any plastic bottle with a nozzle, such as one containing tomato sauce. Clean this very thoroughly, then fill with purified water, or an infusion of *Calendula* flowers, or *Golden Seal*, both of which have an anti-microbial action. Use this bottle to irrigate the perineal and rectal areas, and then pat dry.

⚜ Have no baths, intercourse or vaginal examinations. Don't put your fingers into your vagina to feel what's happening, and use sterile pads to absorb the moisture.

Above all, be guided by your carer as to the appropriate course of action.

Past obstetric history of haemorrhage/retained placenta/prematurity
Good health care prior to and during pregnancy may well reduce the risk associated with these conditions.

Twins (depending on their size)
If twins are very small (less than 2.5 kilos/5½ lbs) and vulnerable they may require immediate medical attention.

Previous injury to uterus

You can heal and strengthen your uterus before labour to reduce the risk of repeat damage or insufficient muscle tone. Nutrients such as zinc and vitamins A and E (for healing), silica (for tissue strength) and calcium and magnesium (for muscle tone) will be important. The herbs to use include *Nettle*, *Raspberry* and *True Unicorn Root*, which are safe to take during pregnancy, or *Blue Cohosh* and *False Unicorn Root* if treatment takes place before conception.

Tumours (eg fibroids) which lie between the baby's head and the birth canal

These may be treated with natural remedies, but many of the herbs which are used for treatment are not appropriate during pregnancy, and treatment would need to be complete before conception.

Failure to progress in first or second stage of labour

To speed up a stalled or ineffective labour, most of the remedies we'll discuss below in the sections on natural induction will be appropriate. They include *Black Cohosh*, *Black Haw*, *Cramp Bark*, *False Unicorn Root*, *Dong Quai*, *Beth Root*, *Mugwort*, *Southernwood* and *Schisandra*. However, if you are using the suggested herbal medicines, instead of a substantial dose every two hours or so, you may need to take a smaller dose every 20–40 minutes. In all cases, be guided by your herbalist.

If your cervix is tight, and isn't dilating, *Evening Primrose* or *Flaxseed* oil, as well as being taken internally at 3000 mg daily (see Chapter 4 for daily dose), can be applied directly to the cervix, as can vitamin E oil. Just prick a hole in the capsules that you normally take orally, and squeeze the contents on to a cotton swab or your finger.

Stress or exhaustion can slow your contractions. If this is the case, get some sleep if you can, or use some of the relaxation ideas in Chapter 7. The sedative nervines such as *Skullcap*, *Valerian*, *Passion-flower*, *Chamomile*, *Catnip* or *Wood Betony* (not all of these are suitable during pregnancy) can also help. If you are impatient and frustrated, try the Bach Flower essence *Impatiens*. This is especially useful if things are actually going well, but you are just in a hurry to get it all over (which is no reason to use these remedies).

Homoeopathic remedies which are specific for this time are:

❧ *Belladonna:* if you are agitated, delirious or hot, with a red face and bloodshot eyes.

❧ *Caulophyllum:* take the '30c' potency dose every two hours, with a maximum of six doses in each 24 hours, and continue until your contractions are regular. If this is not effective, take the '200c' potency every half-hour for two to three doses. This remedy also helps to soften the cervix. It can be taken in the '30c' potency, once a day for 10 days before your due date as a preventative remedy.

❧ *Coffea:* if you are experiencing painful but ineffective contractions.

❧ *Gelsemium:* take the '30c' potency dose every half hour for six to eight doses if *Caulophyllum* is ineffective.

❧ *Gossypium:* if you are experiencing intermittent, relatively painless contractions with little progress, or if you are fatigued.

❧ *Potassium phosphate:* this celloid or tissue salt has a reputation for bringing on an overdue labour.

❧ *Pulsatilla:* if your labour is slow and you feel emotionally vulnerable.

The nutrients which are important for uterine muscle tone are calcium and magnesium. The fastest and easiest way to absorb these minerals is to take the celloids or tissue salts, calcium phosphate and magnesium phosphate, which can be found at your local health food shop—some preparations come as a little pilule that can be dissolved under your tongue.

The remedies for post maturity might be helpful here (see pp. 190–196).

Maternal distress (depending on progress of labour)
In most cases, if you use the remedies we have suggested for stress and pain, you will be able to resolve any problems. However, there are some conditions (for example the pelvic injury that Francesca sustained in a car accident) which are beyond your control, and may require intervention.

Pelvic insufficiency (cephalo-pelvic disproportion)
This problem is often overstated, and if the mother assumes a squatting or semi-squatting position, this will increase the pelvic outlet by approximately 28 per cent.

Conditions which can be managed without medical intervention

Breech presentation
Breech presentation means your baby's head is at the top of your uterus instead of the bottom. Many Caesareans are performed because the obstetrician has no experience of breech delivery. Eighty per cent of breech births can be successfully delivered vaginally, though problems are more likely to be experienced if your baby is very large. The mother should assume the squatting position, as for cephalo-pelvic disproportion to open wide the pelvic outlet.

There are, however, quite a few natural methods for turning a baby in a breech position. These methods can also help with other malpresentations such as transverse lie when your baby is in a horizontal position. There's no need to concern yourself with any of these remedies before the 37th week of your pregnancy, as there is still a chance that your baby will turn head down before the birth.

Acupuncture
One of the most successful and well documented treatments for turning breech babies is moxibustion of the acupuncture point, *Bladder 67*. This point is found at the outside edge of the little toe (on both feet), near the nail. (This point can also be used for stalled labour, but otherwise should *not be used during pregnancy*.) A glowing stick of 'Moxa' (compressed *Mugwort* herb) applies heat to the point. Several studies have confirmed the value of this treatment. One, in Plymouth, UK, gave a 60–65 per cent success rate. Another, a randomised, controlled, clinical trial carried out in Italy, compared 130 first-time mothers carrying breech babies in their 33rd week, with another 130 mothers in the control group. Seventy-five per cent of the babies in the moxibustion group had turned head down by the end of the 35th week, compared to only 48 per cent of those in the control group, and a significant increase in foetal movement was observed.

After this time the mothers were given the option of external manipulation of the baby (see below). Twenty-four women in the control
group and one in the moxibustion group chose this option. The control
group's success rate only rose to 62 per cent, despite this higher level
of intervention.

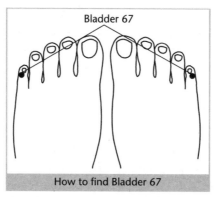

How to find Bladder 67

If you are using moxibustion, the treatment should continue for 15–
20 minutes on each foot, up to ten times daily. Tonifying pressure
(stationary or clockwise pressure for two minutes) on the point may
also be useful. The pressure can be slowly increased as your tolerance
of any discomfort increases. If you press too hard straight away, you
may tense. Pressure that increases gradually can be better tolerated.
Alternatively, a paste of freshly crushed *Ginger* can be applied to each
little toe before retiring. Another study, which compared 133 women
using the *Ginger* paste between 28th and 38th weeks of pregnancy
with a control group of 238 women, found that 42.5 per cent of the
babies in the treatment group turned spontaneously, after just one
treatment, with 77 per cent responding after repeated treatments. In
the control group, only 51.6 per cent of the babies turned before birth.

Homoeopathy
The homoeopathic remedy *Pulsatilla* has a reputation for correcting
malposition. Used in the '30c' potency, you can take a dose three times
daily for up to 10 days, or one dose every two hours, up to a maximum
of six doses, during a single day only. One Adelaide homoeopath,
Thomas Dellman, claims an 80 per cent success rate when this method
is combined with yoga.

Yoga
The inverted yoga poses are traditionally used to help turn a breech

baby, though it's best if you are experienced with these, or are supervised by a qualified teacher. This is particularly important for headstands, and any pregnant woman is likely to need physical support while assuming this position. We've seen it suggested that one way to achieve support is to practise the headstand while fully immersed in water. While we're aware that yoga practitioners can, and do, develop an extraordinary level of breath control, we feel this may be too hazardous for general use!

Other inversions

There are other inverted positions that you can try even if you don't practise yoga. Just make sure you practise an inversion *before* you eat. All these positions take pressure off the uterus, allowing your baby to move easily and turn around. As your baby's head is the heaviest part of his body, gravity will do the work for you, if he is free to move. A slant-board is easy to use at home. Find an old door (we know you've always got one of those kicking around somewhere), a piece of wood strong enough to hold your weight, or even an ironing board. Put one end on the floor and one on your bed, or a chair, so the slant-board tilts at an angle of approximately 45° (see diagram 1). Make sure the set-up is very secure, then lie, head down, for about 10–20 minutes twice daily. Stop if you feel dizzy or experience pain. While you're lying there, gently massage your belly (see Chapter 7) and breathe deeply, as relaxation can also help. You can do this from the twenty-eighth week of your pregnancy, though, as we've said, you needn't be too concerned about malpositions until week 37.

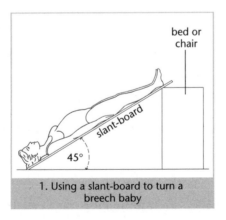

bed or chair

slant-board

45°

1. Using a slant-board to turn a breech baby

The 'Indian Bridge' is another position you can try and this is claimed to have a success rate of 89 per cent. Lie on your back on the floor or a flat surface. Put two or three pillows or cushions, or a beanbag, under your hips and buttocks, and preferably none under your head. If you are really uncomfortable, use a very small cushion for your head, which needs to be lower than your hips (see diagram 2). Bend your knees, with your feet flat on the floor. This position can be practised twice a day, for up to 15 minutes at a time, starting at 30 weeks. It usually takes about three weeks to work.

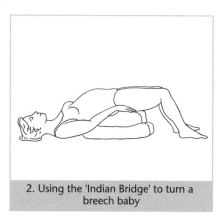

2. Using the 'Indian Bridge' to turn a breech baby

Another position, which some mothers find more comfortable, is to get down on your hands and knees, without letting your thighs touch your belly, and put your head, shoulders and upper chest flat on the floor. Allow your belly to relax, and give your baby room to move (this is 'The Child's Pose'—see the two diagrams, page 100). You can assume this position for 15 minutes, every two hours for five days. As with the other positions, stop if you feel dizzy, seriously uncomfortable or experience any pain.

Relaxation and hypnotherapy

All methods of relaxation are helpful for turning a baby (see Chapter 7). Hypnotherapy has been used successfully, and is valuable if you are finding it difficult to relax on your own. Your therapist can also teach you how to use self-hypnosis. Alternatively, visualise your baby turning head down, or think about his head crowning first. Talk to your baby as you visualise the desired outcome, while lying in one of the inverted positions we've suggested.

External manipulation

A very experienced midwife or obstetrician may be able to turn your baby using external manipulation. This process is called External Cephalic Version (ECV). However there is a risk that the cord may twist around the baby's head as he somersaults, so it is not used routinely. Sometimes a drug is given to relax the uterus, and the baby's heart rate is monitored. If the first attempt is not successful, the approach is abandoned, and the baby is left in the breech position. The success rate isn't high, and though two studies have shown rates of 60 per cent and 45 per cent, the baby will often turn back to his original position.

Twins (depending on their size)

If your twins each weigh more than 2.5 kg (5½ lbs), then they are likely to be robust enough to survive easily once they are born. If, however, they are very large, your labour may be extra demanding. This won't necessarily require intervention, but be prepared.

Mother under 18 years/over 35

Although these age groups are, statistically, at greater risk of complications, this can be greatly reduced if you are well prepared, and you should be confident that you can labour effectively without intervention.

First birth

Statistics again show a high risk of complications in first births, and in some countries only second and subsequent births take place at home. However, as with the risks attached to age, your preparation will be the key to a successful experience.

Anaemia

If you are anaemic, the capacity of the red blood cells to supply oxygen to your body is reduced. Anaemia is common in pregnancy, when the volume of blood increases markedly, and is a problem for both you and your baby. You may feel weak or dizzy, experience palpitations and shortness of breath, and your whole body, including your nail beds, may be very pale. Anaemia will worsen with blood loss, so it's important to treat it well before your due date. If your red blood cell count is low, *Dong Quai* can increase it.

There are three different types of anaemia—iron deficiency, folic acid deficiency (megaloblastic anaemia) and vitamin B12 deficiency (pernicious anaemia). If you followed our dietary recommendations before and throughout your pregnancy, it is unlikely that anaemia will be a problem. However, if you feel excessively tired, a full blood count will tell you if you are anaemic, and blood tests for folate and B12 will detect a grave deficiency. The blood test for iron shows circulating and stored iron (ferritin) levels, and should be performed at the end of each trimester. A satisfactory level for serum ferritin is between 55–65 mcg per litre. See page 79 for appropriate dosages.

If the iron supplement is not organic and chelated, you may suffer from constipation. Furthermore, don't supplement unless the need is proven, since iron can be toxic in excess and also inhibits the absorption of zinc. Folic acid should always be taken with the full range of B-complex vitamins.

Herbal and food sources of iron
- Seaweed (make sure it's organic, since coastal waters can be quite polluted)
- Spinach (but remember that iron from a plant source is not as bio-available as that from meat)
- Red meat (haem-iron is the most easily absorbed)
- *Nettle, Withania, Alfalfa* and *Parsley* (these herbs are rich in iron)

Vitamin C helps you assimilate iron, but dairy products and caffeine inhibit absorption. The celloid or tissue salt ferrum phosphate is an easily assimilated form of iron that ensures rapid uptake. However, parsley should not be eaten in excess during pregnancy (so don't binge on tabouli!).

Herbal and food sources of folic acid
- *Parsley, Dandelion Leaves* and *Watercress* (these can be added to your salads)
- *Nettle* and *Red Raspberry* (these can be drunk as herbal teas)

Herbal and food sources of vitamin B12
- Whole grains and vegetables (only present in very small quantities)
- Nuts and seeds (only present in very small quantities)

- Yoghurt (only present in small quantities)
- Meat (this is the most reliable source)

Vegetarians beware: animal foods, especially meats, are the richest source of this vitamin.

Other therapies

Both reflexology and acupuncture have been shown to correct anaemia. Use stimulation and massage of the reflex points for the spleen and liver. (See the reflexology diagram in Appendix 1.)

Acupuncture was shown in a clinical trial to be as successful as iron supplementation in treating anaemia and low haemoglobin levels. The points used were:

- *Bladder 17*: on either side of the spine, level with the base of the scapula (shoulder-blade).
- *Gall Bladder 39*: four finger widths up (the fourth finger finds the spot), from your ankle bone on the outside of your leg.

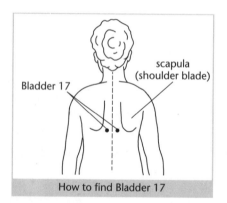

How to find Bladder 17

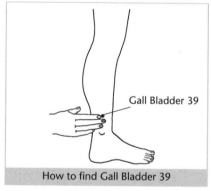

How to find Gall Bladder 39

Stomach 36 was also used in this trial, but this point should not be stimulated in late pregnancy.

You should use tonifying pressure (stationary or clockwise pressure for two minutes) on these points, if you are using self-help acupressure. Alternatively, you could consult an acupuncturist, who might choose different points, depending on your condition and the individual diagnosis.

Irregular contractions

The herbs that will be helpful if your contractions are irregular and spasmodic are mostly the same ones that we recommended earlier for delayed or stalled labour. They include *Black Cohosh*, *Black Haw*, *Cramp Bark*, *False Unicorn Root*, *Dong Quai*, *Beth Root*, *Mugwort*, *Southernwood* and *Schisandra*. Two other herbs that may assist are *Feverfew* and *Mistletoe*. All these should be taken at the dose prescribed by the dispensing herbalist. Nervine herbs can also help if stress or fatigue is part of the problem, as can calcium and magnesium, which will also improve uterine muscle tone.

Lavender and *Mandarin* oils can be massaged on your lower back and belly, or used in a warm bath. As well as those suggested previously, homoeopathic remedies include:

- *Aconitum:* for frequent but irregular contractions.
- *Cocculus:* for spasmodic, irregular pains in the small of the back, especially if you feel exhausted and out of control.
- *Nux vomica:* for inefficient contractions that have almost ceased.

Prolonged labour (if still progressing)

The same remedies can be used as those we recommended for 'Failure to progress' in the previous section. Try to stay relaxed, as tension slows labour down.

Previous Caesarean sections

Vaginal birth is less risky than a repeat Caesarean, and can usually take place at home. You can strengthen your womb with the same nutrients and herbs we suggested for 'Previous injury to uterus' in the previous section.

Oedema

Fluid retention is quite common in late pregnancy, but since it can be a sign of pre-eclampsia, consult your health practitioner if you experience any swelling or bloating. If your feet and lower legs become swollen towards the end of the day, but appear normal by the next morning, the oedema is probably not of great concern. However if swelling is constant; if finger pressure leaves an indentation in your flesh, or if it's present in your face and hands in the morning, it may be a symptom of something more serious. Here's what you can do.

⚹ Drink lots of purified water (two to three litres daily). This 'flushes' out your kidneys and makes them more efficient.

⚹ Exercise regularly.

⚹ Eat plenty of protein.

⚹ Salt your food to taste (use sea or rock salt only and don't salt heavily or routinely).

⚹ Lie on your left side.

⚹ Elevate your feet as often as possible.

⚹ Use diuretic herb teas such as *Dandelion, Cleavers* and *Nettle*. Eat *Dandelion Leaves* in your salad.

⚹ Have a massage of the affected areas.

⚹ Try reflexology when you're having your feet massaged. The points to stimulate are those for the kidneys, bladder and ureters (see Appendix 1 for a diagram showing these points).

⚹ Try the following homoeopathic remedies:

  • *Apis:* especially if the swelling is worse in the late evening and on your right side; if the skin over the affected area looks waxy and transparent; if your urine is scanty or if you have no thirst and are very tired. Take one dose of the '12c' potency in the morning.
  • *Arsenicum album:* especially if you have extreme thirst for small, frequent drinks, are short of breath on exertion, are restless but exhausted or have swelling mainly in your feet and cramps in your calves.
  • *Prunus spinosa:* especially if you have swollen ankles and feet which feel sprained, swollen fingers which itch at the tips, an urgent need to urinate with a slow start to the flow of urine, or a shooting headache.

Postmaturity

As we discussed in Chapter 2, the natural length of a pregnancy is nine lunar months, or 266 days from conception (see Appendix 2), though each pregnancy will have its own pace, and each baby its own rate of development. However, a baby is considered by the medical world to be postmature if the pregnancy extends beyond 42 weeks, though many babies are born quite successfully, with no problems, as late as 44 weeks.

It's not really clear whether the trigger for birth comes from the mother or the child, but it certainly happens, in nearly all cases, when the child and/or mother have reached a natural point of development which is the right time for that baby to be born. Interventions in this process can only rarely be justified in terms of saving lives or major trauma, and are more often the result of a lack of faith in the natural process, or a belief that we need to impose our own sense of 'order' on the 'chaos' of nature.

Scientists are starting to understand that dynamic systems in nature tend to 'self-organisation'—the spontaneous production of self-sustaining patterns or forms—but there is still far too frequently a tendency to want to interfere and control, and a lack of trust in the way natural events unfold. Whereas there are situations where intervention is necessary because something is amiss in the natural progression, the chances are, if you are healthy, your nutritional status is good and you have no pre-existing condition which predisposes you to a difficult birth, that any kind of induction is unnecessary and may indeed have more to do with the convenience of your medical practitioner, who may believe that it is unimportant to let nature take its course. Possible conditions that your medical practitioner might advise as reasons for an induction, other than postmaturity, could include:

- *Prolonged or premature rupture of membranes:* see 'Conditions which may require medical management'. Nutritional deficiencies are a major cause of this condition (see Chapter 4), and are less likely to occur if you've been eating and supplementing well, before and during your pregnancy.

- *Uncontrolled high blood pressure:* which could progress to pre-eclampsia. Luckily there are also preventative and curative natural remedies for this condition (see pages 163–166).

- *Genital herpes:* even if in remission, to avoid an acute episode being triggered by labour. This, too, can be prevented and treated with natural remedies (see pages 167–170).

- *Previous delivery of a baby over 4 kg:* as subsequent babies are often larger, this is anticipation of problems with delivery if the baby grows to his full birth weight.

Good preconception and pregnancy health care should, luckily, avoid unnecessary inductions for these reasons. It's certainly true, however, that the most common purpose of an induction is to prevent problems with the placenta, which is more likely after 42 weeks. It is important to remember that, unless you know exactly when you conceived (as you will if you were practising Natural Fertility Management and monitoring your cycle), your due dates will have been calculated from your last menstrual period, a practise which results in at least 50 per cent of all babies spontaneously arriving after their calculated due date. However, with accurate dates, fewer than two per cent of babies are really more than two weeks overdue.

Once you are 10 days overdue, it's time to start monitoring your baby's activity (through a kick-chart) and his heartbeat. A kick-chart can be drawn up quite simply. Sit quietly, and count the number of movements your baby makes for four half-hour periods per day, preferably at the same time each day. If the total number of movements is fewer than 10 in one whole day, or there is no foetal movement for three successive half-hour periods, you should contact your medical carer, or a hospital.

Remember, babies need sleep too, so don't be alarmed if he is quiet for a whole half-hour period, as he may sleep for up to a couple of hours at any one time.

The next step may be to monitor baby with a cardiotocograph (CTG), twice weekly. After this, ultrasound may be used to assess the size and weight of your baby, the amount of amniotic fluid, and the ratio between these two.

We strongly recommend that, if possible, you avoid invasive procedures such as ultrasound (now shown to affect a baby's growth and health) and the 'stress' test, when oxytocin is administered to evaluate the reaction of the baby's heart rate to uterine contractions.

If your midwife considers that your pregnancy is still progressing normally, there is no need to panic if your baby is reluctant to put in an appearance, and there is absolutely no justification for inductions where there is no real threat to mother or child. However, once the pregnancy reaches 42 weeks' gestation, your baby's head and shoulders may be getting rather large, and there is a greater risk of malpresentation. The cranial bones will also be harder, and less able to mould as your baby passes down the birth canal. This increases the risk of cephalo-pelvic disproportion (and a harder time for you!). If you feel you have reason to be concerned, there are some natural remedies you can use to speed things up. The advantages of these treatments are that they are less likely to initiate a distressingly intense labour, or to cause a baby to be born before he is ready, though they may kick-start a process that has stalled. (The same remedies can be used to keep labour progressing well once it has started.) Here are some of the things you can try. (Note: some of the methods we suggest, such as nipple stimulation, will help the cervix to ripen and some can only be effective—and should only be used—if the cervix is already ripe and soft.)

Nipple stimulation

Massaging the breasts and stroking the nipples triggers the release of oxytocin into the bloodstream. You can stimulate your own nipples, or your partner can caress and massage them. In one study, women who stimulated their nipples, areolae and breasts for three hours a day from the 39th week were found to be much less likely than the control group to go past their due dates. These women used their fingertips to massage and stimulate the nipple, areola and whole breast for 15 minutes, alternating sides for one hour, three times daily. (We just hope you've got nothing better to do! Akal Khalsa, a Sydney-based midwife who has delivered more than 700 babies at home, says irreverently that all she has ever seen this technique produce is 'sore tits'.)

Nipple stimulation *can* be very effective, but it can also be risky if there is no supervision, since it can lead to very strong contractions. Another form of sexual stimulation that can bring on labour is a slow and sensual bout of love-making, though this must *only* be attempted if your membranes are still intact. If you assume a 'spooning' position, with your partner facing your back, he can reach around and stimulate your breasts at the same time. As the semen, which is rich in natural prostaglandins, soaks into the cervix, it causes the uterus to contract, so deep penetration (though not too abrasive) is helpful.

If either of these methods starts contractions, stop the stimulation during each contraction, and once they are two minutes apart, stop altogether, or things may progress too fast.

Heat, aromatherapy and squatting

Heat can also help to speed things up, so hot baths and showers may be useful. Add some *Lavender* or *Mandarin* to the bath, use these oils to massage your belly, or put them in a burner. Lying flat will slow your labour, so for as long as you can stay awake, stay upright, go for a walk, and assume the squatting position which opens up your pelvis.

Castor oil

Many midwives swear by castor oil. This can be used in two ways, as a compress on your belly, or taken internally as a purgative.

For a compress, saturate a wool or cotton flannel, folded into four, with cold-pressed castor oil. Place directly on the skin of your lower abdomen and cover with a piece of plastic. Apply a hot water bottle or hot-pack over the compress and then a blanket or towel over the top to keep it all in place. Lie on your back for 30–60 minutes and take the opportunity to meditate, listen to music, read, snooze or focus on your thoughts and feelings.

As a purgative the castor oil is taken internally. The traditional remedy is one tablespoonful of castor oil, taken with orange juice, repeated hourly for three doses. Some recipes include vodka. If you feel (we certainly do) that this is a little violent (not to mention toxic), you could perhaps try more gentle laxatives such as *Senna* or *Cascara*.

Acupuncture and reflexology

A qualified acupuncturist, using needles or moxibustion, will give the most effective treatment. For self-help, try using *Bladder 67*, the same point we recommend for turning a breech baby (see diagram p. 183). If you have no access to *Moxa*, use a strong, tonifying pressure on this point and on *Spleen 6* which is four finger widths (the fourth finger finds the spot) above the ankle bone on the inside of your leg, in the small hollow just behind the tibia (see diagram page 134).

You can also try massaging the reflex zones for the pelvis, large intestine, rectum, hypothalamus and pituitary (see the diagrams in Appendix 1, page 279).

Helpful herbs

Most of the following herbs will only work if your cervix is ripe and

your membranes have broken, since they act by stimulating contractions.

- *Blue Cohosh:* if there has been a history of late births, this herb
  can be used after week 37, but only if there are no Braxton-Hicks
  contractions. Otherwise, reserve this herb for an overdue labour.
  If you're overdue, three to eight drops of the fluid extract can be
  taken, in warm water, every hour for up to four hours, or until
  your contractions are regular.

- *Black Cohosh:* this herb also helps to soften the cervix. Use 10
  drops of the fluid extract under the tongue every hour for three to
  four hours, or until the cervix is fully soft and ripe.

- *Golden Seal:* this herb is oxytocic, and will stimulate contractions.

- *Pennyroyal* and *Tansy:* these herbs are traditionally used to bring
  on a period (emmenagogues) and can help to kick-start labour.
  Pennyroyal oil can be used in a burner or inhaled.

- *Southernwood* and *Beth Root:* these herbs are traditionally used
  to speed up and ease labour.

- *Ginger* and *Mugwort:* these are warming herbs, which can help
  to increase uterine circulation.

- *Raspberry* and *Squaw Vine:* these are parturient herbs that help
  all aspects of labour.

- *Schisandra:* this herb has been shown in clinical trials to help
  bring on a delayed labour and increase infrequent or weak
  contractions.

A combination of these herbs can be used. The dosage will depend on
the preparation used and should be set by a dispensing herbalist. The
recommended dose could be taken every two hours for three to four
doses or until labour is established.

Homoeopathic remedies and tissue salts

- *Caulophyllum:* take the '30c' potency dose every two hours, with
  a maximum of six doses in each 24 hours, and continue until your
  contractions are regular. If this is not effective, take the '200c'

potency every half-hour for two to three doses. This remedy also helps to soften the cervix and helps ineffectual or intermittent contractions. It can be taken in the '30c' potency, once a day for 10 days before your due date as a preventative remedy.

- *Gelsemium:* take the '30c' potency dose every half hour for six to eight doses if *Caulophyllum* is ineffective. This remedy is also useful for ineffectual contractions.

- *Potassium phosphate:* this celloid or tissue salt has a reputation for bringing on an overdue labour.

FACING MEDICAL INTERVENTION

If you find yourself having to cope with any of the conditions we've outlined above, and it becomes apparent that natural therapies will not provide all the answers, you'll need to talk with your carer about medical management. The situation will be much easier if you've discussed any possible complications and interventions with your carer and support people well in advance, as it can be difficult when you're in the midst of a situation to make a decision, or communicate your wishes and have them respected. Making a birth plan (as outlined in Chapter 8) and discussing it with your carer is a good start. It may also be helpful if you nominate a spokesperson (your partner/a friend) who can make sure that any situation is managed in a way which is as close to your wishes as possible.

Then, if you choose medical management, or it can't be avoided, induction and Caesarean are the two major interventions you could face. We looked at some of the disadvantages in Chapter 2 (along with some other interventions), but here we'll just give you a few tips on how to cope if they're necessary. As we look at them, you should remember that even if medical intervention is not what you wanted or expected, it doesn't mean that things have gone wrong. After all, the main aim of the game is to get your baby born with minimum harm to you both. This may not always be how you've dreamed of it, and you certainly don't want to compromise those first precious days and weeks with your baby, looking back with a lot of regrets. Once your baby has arrived, all your love and energy will be required to focus on mothering and bonding. If something serious does happen, you will need to bring all your emotional strength to bear on moving forwards, rather than going over what might have been.

Induction

Medical methods of induction include:

* *Prostaglandin pessaries*, which have the advantage of leaving you free of any encumbrances such as drips. The pessaries are inserted at night, and again the following morning if labour has not begun by then.

* *Artificial rupture of the membranes*, which allows the baby's head to press directly against the cervix, causing uterine contractions. This process usually occurs, naturally, at some point during labour. The disadvantages of this method are that it can cause the labour to increase in intensity and speed to a distressing degree, and it creates a high risk of infection. Because of this risk, labour should begin within 24 hours. If this doesn't occur, further methods of induction may need to be employed, such as the administration of oxytocin, though careful observation can sometimes make this unnecessary.

* *Oxytocin drips* stimulate labour, often resulting in stronger, longer, more frequent and more painful contractions. The drip will also inhibit movement, so if, despite your best laid plans you end up in this situation, make sure the tube is long enough to give you as much leeway as possible to move around. One possible major problem with this method of induction is that as the strong contractions inhibit the blood flow to the uterus, there may be ill-effects for the baby. The intensity of the labour will also increase the likelihood of the use of painkillers. Even though there is an 80 per cent likelihood that strong contractions will be experienced, there may be little progress in the dilation of the cervix for many hours, which may result in a Caesarean section being advised. It may be advisable to negotiate with your carer not to start labour if the cervix is unfavourable (long, closed and firm).

Caesarean sections

The most common medical reason for a Caesarean is lack of progress of the labour, though how and when a labour gets defined as 'prolonged' is somewhat subjective and variable. A Caesarean section can be lifesaving in five per cent of women giving birth, and if you fall into this category, you'll need to make the best of the situation, and also a few choices.

If the Caesarean section is inevitable (or planned because of some pre-existing condition), an epidural is preferable to a full anaesthetic, though if it's an emergency, a general is more common. If you know in advance that you will be having a Caesarean section, you can reduce the possibility of problems associated with the anaesthetic if you:

- use the homoeopathic remedies *Thuja* and *Staphysagria* for a few days before and after the procedure;

- avoid eating foods of the nightshade family (such as eggplant, tomato, capsicum and potato) for several days beforehand, as these can interfere with the breakdown of the drugs in your body.

Liz's story
We've included here some thoughts from our agent, Liz Courtney, who found her cherished birth plans turned on their head, and herself onto her back, when she needed a Caesarean section. However, we are delighted to say that due to her commitment to preconception and pregnancy health care, her son Dakotah is certainly a delightful, bright and healthy 'better baby'. We're grateful to her for sharing her thoughts. Liz now knows that understanding what happens when you have a Caesarean and what to expect afterwards is very important. It would be a good idea to have discussed these options, and your preferences, with your caregivers before the birth.

- On arrival in the operating theatre there is a lot of activity around you. Blood samples will be taken and you'll be required to take a shower and scrub down your belly with a special disinfectant. You'll be shaved as well and then you'll be given a pre-op injection.

✻ Your partner can be with you, but he'll need to wear a gown. He can hold your hand when the epidural needle is inserted.

✻ If you choose an epidural, you'll be awake during the operation, and much better able to hold and respond to your baby. Alternatively, you can choose to have the procedure carried out under general anaesthetic, in which case you'll be out for the count, and much less able to bond with and nurse your baby. There is also a greater possibility of ill effects for the baby if you opt for a general anaesthetic.

✻ During the procedure, the anaesthetist will sit by your side and can administer more anaesthetic if it becomes necessary.

✻ Your partner can watch the procedure, although usually the site of the incision will be screened from your view, but as soon as the baby is lifted out, the curtain will be removed.

✻ The operation usually takes between 15–20 minutes. Your partner can ask to have the baby put straight into his arms and then, together, you can see him for the first time. If your baby's well, you might be able to extend this first contact.

✻ Your baby will then be taken away for weighing and assessment. It may not be possible to avoid this part of the procedure, as it would be if you'd had an uncomplicated vaginal birth, so it's important that your partner goes with the baby—he can carry him if there are no problems.

✻ You'll have to stay quiet while you're stitched up. You'll then be taken to the post-op area for observation. If there are no complications, you'll then be taken back to your room.

✻ As soon as your baby is back in your arms, you'll be encouraged to nurse him. You might find this uncomfortable because your wound won't allow you to hold him in the normal 'en face' position, but the midwives will show you an alternative way to feed. Nursing will start the flow of colostrum, and it's important that you feed on demand, even if you're feeling 'out of it'. Your baby's sucking will stimulate the production of certain hormones that will actually help you to feel better.

✻ The epidural will remain in place for 24–48 hours, so that analgesic can be administered when necessary. You'll feel the pain as a searing, burning sensation inside you when it wears off, so don't be afraid to tell the staff when this happens. It's better for you to be free of any discomfort and relating well to your baby, than stoically bearing the pain.

- The drugs in your blood stream aren't directly absorbed into your breast milk, but must rely on an active transport system, so your baby gets only the minimal amount of medication.

- It's important that your partner is there to help you wherever possible. You'll need lots of assistance, so don't be afraid to ask for it.

- It's also important to keep taking your supplements—this will speed the healing, prevent any infection, and will also help your body to metabolise and excrete the drugs.

- The day after the birth you'll be helped to the shower. This can be challenging, and you should be prepared to feel a bit weak and dizzy. Putting your head between your knees for a few moments can help you to retain your equilibrium, if you are able to perform this feat so soon after major abdominal surgery.

- Breastfeeding may be tricky at first—you may need to feed your baby twin style. This means he will lie along your side with his feet towards your back, but in a few weeks you will be able to assume the normal position.

- Your stitches are usually removed on about day 5, though this could be as late as day 6–8. This is usually the hardest day after a Caesarean. You might feel a bit weepy—this is common and is a delayed reaction. If your zinc status was adequate before the birth, you shouldn't be too troubled by any hint of postnatal depression, but you now have to deal with the disappointment of missing out on a natural birth.

- You should try to walk every day. Take it slowly at first and don't overdo things—it's not a competition.

- For the first few days, your diet should be light, easily digested foods. Your bowels might take a few days to get working again, but plenty of water (and some high-fibre drinks) can help.

- You'll also experience a lot of wind in the first few days. This is normal after the type of procedure you've just undergone.

- About six weeks after the birth, you should begin to strengthen the area that was cut. Yoga is great for doing this. If you start too early, there is a risk that the wound will separate.

- Don't try lifting anything heavier than the baby in the first six weeks, and pay close attention to this advice. If you strain too hard, you could find your wound takes a lot longer to heal, and that will delay your recovery and your return to full mobility. You will also place yourself at risk of haemorrhage or uterine prolapse.

- To get up from a lying down position, you should turn on your side, push yourself up with your hands, swing your legs over the side of the bed and get up that way. This will allow your tummy muscles time to heal.

- It's good if you can have someone with you on a full time basis during these weeks. You'll need help to lift your baby up and, if you're trying to manage alone, you might tend to leave him in his cot. However, since you missed out on some of the benefits of a natural birth, it's important that you spend as much time in close contact with your baby as possible.

- Don't be afraid to accept whatever help is offered—meals cooked, washing done, house cleaned. Your focus needs to be on making a speedy recovery and on being close to your baby, so the more help you can get, the better it will be for both of you.

- See Chapter 12 for more recovery remedies.

BE PREPARED FOR THE UNEXPECTED

If, like Liz, you didn't get the birth you wanted or expected, you'll find considerable comfort if you accept that there is a greater hand at work in all our lives. It might sometimes be difficult to accept the wisdom of that hand, but if you just remember that the Universe always gives you what you *need*, even if this is not necessarily what you *want*, you will learn and gain something from every single experience that life presents to you.

When you are at ease with this fact, you are really able to get on with the job in hand. It's not very productive to dwell on what might have been, or on the reasons why things went the way they did. It's not smart to look for someone to blame, nor is it clever for you to burden yourself with guilt. Instead, it's important that you focus on all the positive things that you have done, and get on with the very important task of nurturing your baby. If you know that there were ways in which you could have been better prepared, things which could have been managed differently, or perhaps it was simply that omnipotent hand teaching you a little wisdom and humility—accept it, learn from it, and *let it go*.

As Francesca's experiences, which are recounted in the Foreword, show, if you trust your caregivers to make the choices that you prefer; if you feel as involved as possible in all the decisions that are made; if you have prepared yourself with information and good support people; and if you go into your birthing experience with an open mind, you'll be able to flow with whatever occurs, and come through it all knowing that you and your baby had the best birth possible, just as you will go on to be the best mother possible (and allow yourself to be human and make mistakes!).

Even when the birth seems to have gone completely 'to plan', there may still be a few surprises. Janette knows this only too well. She hopes that her little story of the birth of her second son will show you that things can go unexpectedly awry.

With the birth of Michael, Jan had a short but intense labour at home. Michael was born after a second stage of eight minutes, he scored APGAR 9 and 10, the midwife had enjoyed a cup of tea with the new father and had headed home for some sleep. Jan got into bed to nurse her newborn son and all seemed absolutely fine. Then about five hours after the birth, Michael's breathing rate became very rapid. A back-up midwife was called, the neonatal flying squad followed close on her heels and the next 48 hours saw this baby undergoing all the high-tech investigations and monitoring that Jan had wanted so much to avoid. Fortunately, the good start that he had saw him dismissed in a relatively short time with a diagnosis of 'inhaled vernix'. This was just one of those chance things for which nobody can really prepare but which made Jan aware that birth, indeed like all of life, always contains the unexpected element, and that, realistically, you need to be prepared for any eventuality.

Natural or medical management for your baby?

The birth of your baby is the culmination of many months of preparation, care, waiting, and planning. You will have invested a considerable amount of time and effort in being as healthy as you possibly can so that your baby will enjoy the same good health. You'll have spent a good deal of time learning about what to expect at the birth, and how to get the most out of the experience.

But there are several procedures that are a routine part of postpartum care for your baby which you need to be familiar with as well. These can affect your baby's health and wellbeing, so it's important that you're aware of what's involved, and decide in advance how you feel about each. Having taken great pains to make sure that your baby gets off to the best possible start, you don't want to undo some of that good work by being unprepared or uninformed about these procedures.

APGAR SCORE

This is the method by which the condition of a newborn baby is evaluated.

Five vital signs are assessed at 60 seconds and again at five minutes after the birth. A best possible score of 2 is given for each; a score of 1 is OK but not optimal, and a score of 0 is given if the response is absent. A healthy baby will initially score between 7 and 10, and usually achieve a score of 10 at the five minute assessment. The signs noted are:

- A—appearance (colour)
- P—pulse
- G—grimace (This is the annoyed response to suctioning or stroking the sole of the foot. We hope your baby won't need suctioning, but will respond to foot stroking.)
- A—activity (The baby who has had an unmedicated birth may be quite calm, there may be no protests to assess, and you may not want to stimulate any. It's a shame to disturb that calm by trying to elicit this response by provoking the baby. However even a relaxed baby will make some involuntary uncoordinated movements and you can observe these.)
- R—respiration (breathing)

NEWBORN SCREENING (FORMERLY CALLED GUTHRIE HEEL PRICK TEST)

This is a diagnostic test for a condition known as phenylketonuria (PKU), a metabolic disorder that can lead to severe mental retardation. But if it is diagnosed early and an appropriate diet implemented, the ill effects can be completely avoided. Newborn Screening also checks for hypothyroidism, galactosaemia and cystic fibrosis. To perform the test, your baby's heel will be pricked and three drops of blood collected. This small amount of blood is necessary to make a diagnosis. The test is quite stressful for your baby and it's usually carried out away from your sight and hearing, so that you won't be distressed. While it's certainly normal for you to be upset by your baby's distress, it will be less traumatic for him if you hold him in your arms while the procedure is performed, and cuddle and nurse him immediately afterwards.

VITAMIN K

It is now routine practice in hospitals to administer vitamin K, orally or through intra-muscular injection, to every newborn baby. Vitamin K is a fat-soluble vitamin and is required for the liver to form prothrombin and proconvertin, which are factors involved in the process of blood clotting and which prevent haemorrhage as well as being involved in healthy bone mineralisation. Vitamin K is normally formed by bacteria in the intestines; however a newborn infant is not able to produce it as his intestinal flora is not yet fully established, and he is born with only a few days' supply, which is inherited from his mother.

The maternal supply of vitamin K will be greater if the mother has a healthy gut and a diet rich in foods that provide vitamin K, though it doesn't easily cross the placental barrier. A few days after birth, there will be a decrease of vitamin K in the baby, whose own blood clotting mechanisms will not be established for about eight days. So the newborn has a prolonged clotting time for the first week of life, and this can lead to a potential risk of Vitamin K Deficiency Bleeding (VKDB) or Haemorrhagic Disease of the Newborn (HDN).

Even small haemorrhages can be serious, such as those from the gastrointestinal tract which manifest as nose bleeds, bleeding from the bowel or the vomiting of blood, bleeding from the stump of the umbilical cord, or from a circumcised penis. Bleeding into the brain can be fatal. The occurrence of these haemorrhages is highest in the fourth to sixth weeks of life, and can continue up to the 26th week, though the risk of brain haemorrhage is very slight.

The practice of giving vitamin K to newborn babies started in the 1950s when it was administered only to those infants considered at high risk. Gradually it became routine for all babies to have an injection. However, there are questions and concerns that have been raised about its safety, especially if given through injection. One study, reported in the *British Medical Journal*, compared vitamin K shots with oral administration. The researchers were surprised to find that bleeding was rare even when *no* vitamin K was given, and concluded that usual methods of measurement (which show widespread deficiency) might be insufficient. They also concluded that the risk of brain haemorrhage was very slight (one in ten thousand).

Another two studies carried out in Bristol, England linked vitamin K injections to the risk of childhood leukaemia being doubled. The researchers in one of these studies suggested that the intra-muscular dose (of 1 mg) should be restricted to babies at high risk of HDN, with other babies receiving the same dose orally. Their findings are controversial, but they assessed the risk of the development of leukaemia to one in five hundred, whereas the risk of HDN is only one in ten thousand.

Other concerns are raised by the findings in some animal studies that chromosomes break up after a vitamin K injection, and the fact that, following an injection, a baby's body may contain up to five thousand times the normal level of the vitamin. Oral administration does not appear to result in such an extreme overdose, but, since vitamin K is a fat-soluble vitamin, it should not be given routinely in high doses unless there is a proven need. Since infants are not screened prior to being given vitamin K, it cannot be established that their bodies require it.

All of this raises the question as to whether it is the vitamin K that can cause these problems, whether it is the synthetic form of the vitamin that is used, or whether it is the injection itself. One article in the *British Medical Journal* suggested that there may in fact be a biological advantage to vitamin K deficiency in early infancy, and a possible symbiotic action with breastfeeding.

Despite this, orthodox opinion is still that vitamin K deficiency is abnormal and constitutes a risk to the baby. Little credence is given, in most medical circles, to the idea that it may be a normal and natural physiological phenomenon. Indeed, if not, why is there such a low incidence of HDN? Remember, the risk is only one in ten thousand if vitamin K is *not* administered.

Although the incidence of HDN has decreased since vitamin K has been given routinely, there are other factors that may explain this. Early studies linking this decrease with routine injections used poor populations as the study group, so dietary deficiencies and high rates of infection may have contributed to the then higher incidence of the disease. It is not known if vitamin K is the only causative factor for HDN and it is possible, for example, that viruses passed through the placental barrier might affect liver function and intestinal absorption in the baby (viruses have a natural affinity with the liver and the mucous membranes).

It's also true that breastfeeding has been widely re-established over the same period, and may have contributed to the improving rate. Colostrum is high in vitamin K, though breast milk has less, and the baby receives a plentiful supply in the first days of suckling. To increase your own levels, you need to eat foods that are rich in vitamin K such as broccoli, brussels sprouts, cabbage, green beans, kale, parsley, alfalfa, spinach, lettuce, brown rice, egg yolks, meat and soy beans (see table). Some herbs are also very rich in vitamin K, and you can drink two cups daily of *Raspberry Leaves, Alfalfa, Rose Hip* and *Nettle* teas in the last six weeks of pregnancy. You, the mother, also need to be protected by this vitamin from risk of haemorrhage during birth, and the herbs useful for postpartum bleeding (see also Chapter 9) include *Shepherd's Purse*, which is high in vitamin K.

Vitamin K content of selected foods (mcg/100 g)

Kale	750
Parsley	700
Spinach	350
Broccoli	200
Brussels sprouts	200
Cabbage	50–175
Green beans	40

Since gastric upsets can interfere with vitamin K production, they should be treated promptly, and since the vitamin is fat-soluble, good oils, such as olive (cold-pressed) and essential fatty acids from fish and evening primrose oil should be included in your diet. Some mothers with low levels are given vitamin K injections prior to birth, but this can be easily avoided by following these dietary guidelines. vitamin K supplements should not be taken, as they may affect blood clotting prior to birth.

Since baby formulas are fortified with vitamin K, bottle-fed babies may have an even lower incidence of HDN, and some authorities have been concerned about the risks of full breastfeeding, despite the obvious advantages. However, a World Health Organisation report shows that where babies are deprived of colostrum, the risk is greater than in artificially-fed babies, unless vitamin K is provided soon after birth.

So do you or don't you let your baby receive vitamin K? And, if so, do you choose for it to be administered orally or through injection? It seems clear that delivery through injection should be limited to those babies who are at high risk of HDN (see the table below and also Chapter 12 for treatments for trauma and injury to the baby). Many hospitals now use oral administration routinely, though there is some dispute as to whether this gives equal protection. The problems with oral administration are that the baby may spit or vomit it out, and that absorption may not be as effective. The dose given by injection is 1 mg, and the same dose is used orally, despite these concerns. As a result, some findings are that the oral dose only gives partial protection, preventing approximately 75 per cent of all cases of HDN. Other findings are that it gives equal protection. Only you, in consultation with your caregivers, can make the final choice.

Conditions which place babies at high risk of HDN
(Haemorrhagic Disease of the Newborn)

Forceps delivery (injury more likely)

Caesarean section (injury more likely)

Significant bruising or bleeding

Circumcision (see our thoughts in the text)

Prematurity

Low birth weight

Surgical procedures

Inadequate feeding

Antibiotic treatment

Treatment of mother (during pregnancy) with:

• anticoagulants

• phenobarbitone

• phenytoin

CIRCUMCISION

Circumcision is the surgical removal of the foreskin that covers the head of the penis. Since a baby's foreskin is not retractable at birth, the procedure involves separating the foreskin from the glans of the penis by forcefully tearing the two layers of skin apart and then removing the outer layer. Until relatively recently, most baby boys, within a few days of their birth, were subjected to this barbarity without the benefit of anaesthetic.

The origins of male (and female) circumcision are lost in the mists of time. Circumcision may have been an initiation or fertility rite, it may have been seen as a form of purification, or it may have been a torture inflicted on enemies. However, with the exception of the Jewish race and the medical profession, very few peoples have ever inflicted circumcision on newborns.

Our modern Western enthusiasm for infant circumcision stems from Victorian times when it was felt that young boys with an intact foreskin would learn to masturbate when they were washing themselves. Since masturbation was thought to be responsible for a variety of diseases, including insanity, the medical practitioners of the time reasoned that it made sense to remove the cause of the problem. Since the 1800s there have been numerous attempts to rationalise this procedure which had such very dubious origins. It has been claimed that circumcision prevents penile and cervical cancers and the spread of venereal disease, but all these theories have been totally discredited. The claim that a circumcised penis is easier to keep clean is like advocating tooth extraction as a preferred alternative to brushing.

Very early reports of circumcisions performed on an infant mentioned the great trauma inflicted. The rather misguided belief that babies felt no pain due to their immature nervous systems came much later, along with bottle feeding, rigid schedules for the newborn and other similarly insensitive practices. The fact that many infants lapse into a semi-coma after circumcision probably fueled this totally erroneous belief. During circumcision, the baby's pulse rate, breathing rate and cortisol (stress hormone) levels rise hugely and deep sleep or coma is the shock reaction by which they cope with a very traumatic experience. Recently, for the first time, and reversing previous pronouncements, the American Academy of Paediatrics acknowledged that pain relief is essential for neonatal circumcision.

Apart from the fact that as a medical procedure it has no known therapeutic or prophylactic value, circumcision can be dangerous and can lead to all sorts of complications. One of these, known as meatal ulceration, occurs when the unprotected glans is burned by the baby's urine. Far more serious side effects include haemorrhage, keloid scars, cysts and infections, with some, such as gangrene, leading to complete loss of the penis and testicles. To add insult to injury, circumcision results in the destruction of the hygienic and immunological properties of the intact penis. The psychological effects of circumcision may be just as profound and long-lasting.

Fortunately, circumcision is no longer performed routinely and the Australian College of Paediatrics actively discourages the procedure. There is also a very low rate of circumcision in Europe, although in the United States, the procedure has been widely performed until recently, when the American Academy of Paediatrics reversed its previous position. It is an interesting fact that the USA has the highest number of sexually active circumcised males and the highest rates of genital cancers, STDs and AIDS of any first world nation. Despite the fact that Australian families are now discouraged from circumcising their infants, and despite the fact that 85 per cent of the world's population is not circumcised, some parents still actively choose this elective procedure.

If you feel that your son should look like his circumcised father, you can rest assured that he will accept the differences readily when he is old enough. A simple explanation is all that is required: *'It was once considered healthy to cut off the foreskin, but since your Dad was born, we've learned that isn't the case.'* If you're in any doubt about how your sons will react, you should talk to families who have both circumcised and non-circumcised members and be reassured that there are no problems.

You may have heard of boys whose foreskin did not retract as they got older. This retraction usually occurs quite naturally, although the age at which it happens will vary. Phimosis, which is the name given to the condition of a non-retractable foreskin, sometimes persists into adulthood. It rarely causes problems and circumcision is not necessary to correct the condition.

If you're worried about cleanliness or possible infection, external washing with soap and water is all that your baby boy's penis requires. In fact the circumcised penis is more prone to infection in the first years of life than the uncircumcised penis. Once the foreskin is retractable (and you should never force or try to hurry this), it's a perfectly simple matter to show your son how to wash his penis properly. Just remember that the glans is an *internal organ* and the foreskin is there to cover it and protect it. The foreskin represents about one third of the penile sensitive area, so its removal will significantly reduce the pleasure your son will experience when he's making love and a circumcised penis may result in more trauma to the vagina.

To sum it up, your son's foreskin is a normal, healthy and necessary part of his body and he has a right to a sound, whole body. It is a violation of his rights as a human being if you remove part of his body without his consent. If family members or friends question your decision not to circumcise, you can simply tell them that it is no business of theirs! Fortunately, circumcision is not performed on infant females, and has never been a routine medical procedure in the West. However, we find the fact that it is performed at all, and for equally spurious reasons, as equally abhorrent as male genital mutilation.

Looking back, it is frightening to think of the stress and pain which has been inflicted on newborn males in the interests of so-called cleanliness or 'So he'll look like his father'. Frightening too, that such a widely and routinely practised procedure had its origins in such suspect science. While on the subject of routine practices of dubious origins, and suspect science, we come to the topic of immunisation.

IMMUNISATION

Since immunisation is not performed in the immediate postpartum period, this book is not really the appropriate forum for a lengthy discussion of this very emotive issue. However, the following paragraph will at least set you thinking. Then we'll be back in our next book *The Natural Way to Better Breastfeeding and Beyond* to discuss this issue and the natural alternatives to immunisation more thoroughly.

In the meantime, you can easily do your own research on the side effects of childhood immunisation programs—we've listed some good books in Recommended Reading, or if you're connected to the Internet, you can simply type in 'vaccine injury' and you'll find more than you really need to know. You'll see that anaphylaxis, anaphylactic shock, encephalopathy, residual seizure disorder, seizure and convulsion, brachial neuritis, chronic arthritis, thrombocytopenic purpura, paralytic polio, vaccine-strain polio viral infection, vaccine-strain measles viral infection and early onset Hib type disease are some of the conditions listed on the web site. You'll also learn that a little known program—The National Vaccine Injury Compensation Program (VICP)—was begun about 10 years ago. About 5300 claims have been filed so far and the program has awarded $900 million to 1300 families whose children have been damaged by vaccination. Certainly food for thought, and enough to send you off to look beyond the orthodox medical dogma which makes very little mention of anything more than the safety and the (perceived) benefits of immunisation.

We believe, as do all practitioners of natural and holistic medicine, that a strong and robust immune system is what your baby needs, so that he can effectively deal with viral and other diseases with which he may come in contact. The best way to ensure this for your child is through good nutrition, and using natural medicines to help him through any threat to his good health.

When something goes wrong

Although we've emphasised strongly how desirable and necessary it is for you to have trust in your body to give birth easily to a healthy child, very occasionally something does go seriously wrong and can affect the health, or even the life, of your child.

If you've read our previous books *The Natural Way to Better Babies* and *The Natural Way to a Better Pregnancy*, and have put in place comprehensive preconception and pregnancy health care, then the chance of this will be greatly reduced. But if the worst does happen, here are some things you may feel, and some suggestions for what may help you through such a devastating experience.

PERINATAL DEATH

Perinatal death means death around the time of birth and includes stillbirth and neonatal death. A baby is stillborn if he is born dead, and does not breathe or show evidence of life after 20 weeks of pregnancy (or if the baby weighs more than 400 grams). Before this time, the death of a baby or foetus is called a miscarriage. A neonatal death is that of a live-born infant within 28 days of birth.

Perinatal death is rare, occurring in less than one per cent of births, but if this happens to your baby, statistics will be little comfort. Such a death is undoubtedly one of the most devastating experiences you will ever have to face, and the pain you feel will be intense. However, there are choices to be made, and how you choose to act will make considerable difference to how well you move through, and recover from, this loss.

If your baby's death occurred in the womb, you will have to choose between giving birth and undergoing a Caesarean. While you may not feel able to cope with a full labour as well as your grief, to do so can bring a sense of completion, and gives you a greater chance to identify as a mother.

Although you may be tempted to hide away and ask others to make all the necessary arrangements, mourning and grieving will be much more difficult if you haven't acknowledged and said goodbye to your baby. You must hold and touch him. Even if there is some malformation, you will still feel love and tenderness for this child, and holding him will make the events more real and therefore easier to deal with. You must name your baby. You need to be able to remember him by name. A naming ritual, christening or baptism can be part of the rites you perform at this time. You will also need to register his death and have a funeral, which you should attend. You may want to plant a tree in memory, or create a gravesite that you can visit. It may be helpful, later on, to have a photo to remember your child by. Though family and friends may offer to remove your baby clothes, cradle and other paraphernalia from your home, it will probably, in the long term, be more helpful if you put these away yourself. Then they can be re-dedicated if you choose to conceive another child.

Though you may be offered sedation, try to avoid any medication that will blur the experience for you, as this will delay grieving and healing. The flower essences may be helpful, as they give you strength but help you retain clarity. *Rescue Remedy*, which is a combination of *Star of Bethlehem* (for shock); *Impatiens* (for mental tension); *Cherry Plum* (for desperation); *Clematis* (for withdrawal); and *Rock Rose* (for terror), can be used freely, as often as required, or added to drinking water. Four drops under the tongue, and held in the mouth for a few moments, can be taken four times daily, or as frequently as every five or ten minutes. Other flower essences you might find helpful could include:

- *Agrimony* (for mental torture behind a 'brave face')
- *Crab Apple* (for feeling your body has let you down)
- *Honeysuckle* (for clinging to what might have been)
- *Mustard* (for deep depression)
- *Olive* (for exhaustion)
- *Pine* (for guilt)
- *Red Chestnut* (for anxiety for others)
- *Sweet Chestnut* (for extreme anguish and bereavement)
- *White Chestnut* (for unwanted thoughts that prey on your mind)

Lastly, cry as often as you need to.

Why has this happened?

Often no tangible cause is found for stillbirth, though studies are now showing clearly that in areas close to sources of environmental pollution, there is an increased rate of perinatal death. If you are thinking of planning another conception soon, you will feel much more confident of a successful outcome if you practise preconception and pregnancy health care (see our books *The Natural Way to Better Babies* and *The Natural Way to a Better Pregnancy* listed in Recommended Reading). It's also evident that babies of couples who have experienced fertility problems, especially where these problems have been solved by recourse to assisted reproductive technology, are more likely to suffer perinatal death. So it's preferable to seek out natural remedies if you have difficulty conceiving.

Often your first warning that something may be wrong is when your baby ceases to move. If this happens, you should seek help immediately. Another warning sign is if you lose weight suddenly (due to the absorption of the amniotic fluid). If this occurs, you should also seek advice, though it may be too late to save the baby. One identifiable and common problem is an insufficiently healthy placenta, which cannot deliver an adequate supply of oxygen and nutrients to your child, or that separates from the uterus. Again, we feel that good, natural health care before and during pregnancy can go a long way to preventing this. Uncontrolled Rhesus disease is another possible cause—this should be medically monitored.

Help is available

You may need to seek help outside your family to assist you through the mourning and grieving processes, as your partner, children, parents and siblings will also be experiencing loss and intense sadness. As much as you may need to cling to each other, you may find professional help gives invaluable extra support.

SANDS, the Stillbirth and Neonatal Death Support group, grief counsellors, spiritual groups, or your health practitioner can all help you deal with your bereavement. Although you may feel a need to withdraw, you will also have a huge range of confusing emotions to deal with. Shock, anger, frustration, despair, depression, guilt, inadequacy and self-loathing may all accompany the grief, extreme sadness and loss you feel. There are ways of helping you to express these emotions and move through them—it's easy to become 'stuck' if you try to cope on your own.

A remedy for many bereaved parents is to conceive again as quickly as possible. Although this can be very positive, you need to give yourself time to mourn and time to replenish your nutritional status. This will be depleted after your pregnancy and further depleted by the stress of your loss. You may also need time to work through your fear of a repeat experience, which many people find inhibits conception.

You won't ever forget the baby you lost, but you need to remember that it is still possible for you to move on to, and grow towards, future positive experiences.

Relationship problems

The great distress and intense emotional states that follow perinatal death can affect your relationships with your family and friends, just when you are most in need of their support. You may find it too painful to talk about what you've been through, or there may be blame, guilt, resentment or a sense of failure that makes good communication difficult. You and your partner both need support, but you may express your feelings very differently. This, again, can be a time when professional support can be invaluable, if you are too upset to help each other.

Remember that your other children, if you have any, will also be distressed. You may be feeling resentful of them, or just too irritable to cope well, at the very time when they are also confused and sad. They may feel guilty that they are alive and their sibling is dead, or angry that the baby has caused so much distress to the family. They need to be able to express these feelings, without being told they are inappropriate. If you feel unable to give them this support, let them find it with other friends or family members to whom they feel close.

Above all, try to recognise if, and when, you simply can't cope, and seek professional help.

POSTNATAL DEPRESSION

Although perinatal death is an experience which may only affect a very small proportion of parents, it is increasingly common for new mothers to suffer from postnatal depression, which can also be extremely debilitating and traumatic. This condition doesn't only affect mothers who have experienced trauma, though this can be a contributing factor, and it can also affect fathers. It should not be confused with the 'Baby Blues' (see below) which commonly occur soon after birth—though the two conditions may occur as a continuum—or with sleep deprivation, though this may also be one of the factors contributing to postnatal depression. It is not usually finally diagnosed until about six weeks after birth, though it may have been present well before this.

It is a particular form of stress and may need to be treated a little differently from the stresses of late pregnancy and childbirth that we have discussed already. Our thanks go to Anna Brennan, a naturopath who has worked with Francesca at the Jocelyn Centre, for her helpful thoughts and research on this topic.

The onset and duration of postnatal depression can vary widely, with the symptoms becoming obvious at any time in the first year after birth, though the first twelve weeks are the period of highest risk. It can last anything from a few weeks to two or three years, though, take heart, this is rare. If symptoms are of short duration, the probability is that you are suffering from the 'Baby Blues', but if they persist beyond two or three weeks, you should seek professional help. Postnatal depression affects between 15–20 per cent of mothers (and up to 10 per cent of fathers). It can occur after the birth of any child, not just the first, though if you have a history of previous bouts of postnatal depression you may be more likely to experience it with subsequent births. Its causes are multi-factorial, as we shall see, and the depression and anxiety experienced can range from mild to severe. Although it is quite normal for most mothers to experience some of the symptoms of postnatal depression at least occasionally, when they start to become frequent, more intense and more long-term, you may need help.

Baby Blues

The 'Baby Blues' are sometimes called the 'Three-Day Baby Blues' and indeed occur at about the third day after birth, when the milk comes in. However, they can surprise you at any time up to 10 days postpartum. They occur in 80 per cent of all mothers, and are due to the massive drop in the hormones oestrogen and progesterone that takes place after birth. In three days or so, these return to pre-pregnancy levels. Since your hormones during pregnancy build slowly over many months to levels that are up to fifty times higher than they were before conception, this sudden drop is indeed massive.

Other factors contribute to the 'Baby Blues'. The experience is characterised by tearfulness and uncontrollable bouts of crying, with feelings of confusion, anxiety, vulnerability, uncertainty, lack of confidence and irritability. In fact, you may suddenly feel completely overwhelmed by the responsibilities of motherhood, worried about your feelings (or lack of) towards your baby, and quite flat after the huge build-up to and excitement of the birth itself. Exhaustion from the rigours of giving birth and sleep deprivation also play a part, and your mood won't be helped if you are experiencing after-pains, sore breasts or nipples, or tenderness in the belly or perineum after a Caesarean or an episiotomy.

If this all sounds a bit gloomy, don't despair—the 'Baby Blues' usually only last 24–48 hours, and in our experience are a non-event with mothers who have taken care of their health and nutritional status before and during pregnancy. They are also less likely if you have had a homebirth or a birth in which you were an active participant in control of the experience, and if the birth took place in a loving and supportive environment with no separation from your baby afterwards. If you are in hospital, and you find the environment depressing, it may be time to check out (as long as you have somewhere to go where you will be supported and cared for). But if you need to stay, it may be helpful to talk to the other new mums about your, and their, feelings. Very early discharge (4–8 hours after birth) has been shown to contribute to postnatal depression, so be sure you're ready to go and it's not a case of 'out of the frying pan and into the fire'. If you are at home, you may need to discourage visitors, so you can get enough sleep, rest and relaxation. All the remedies we'll suggest for postnatal depression may also help you at this time, though a good cry may be enough! If you are worried about your lack of feelings for your baby, or your inadequacy as a mother, be patient. Take one day at a time, and let it all fall into place at its own pace.

Postpartum psychosis

Rarely, in about 0.01–0.02 per cent of women (that is, 1–2 in 1000), a serious depressive condition develops. Postpartum psychosis occurs about two to three weeks after the birth, and will need medical attention, and even hospitalisation. There may be a substantial loss of contact with reality for extended periods of time, with delusions, hallucinations and obsessional behaviour. New mothers suffering from this disorder can hear voices, have suicidal thoughts, have difficulty concentrating, construct grandiose and unrealistic schemes, and experience panic attacks, paranoia and hostility toward their family or their baby. This is not a condition which will respond to the suggested treatments that follow, and must be medically managed.

Symptoms of postnatal depression

Postnatal depression falls somewhere between the 'Baby Blues' and postpartum psychosis. It can certainly be a serious condition, but can usually be managed with lifestyle and natural measures (or prevented similarly by good preconception and pregnancy health care). It might better be called Postnatal Depression and *Anxiety*, or Postnatal Mood Disorder, to encompass the wide range of symptoms which can vary considerably in severity and duration. However, it is a very real condition, not simply put on for sympathy, as some friends and relatives may suspect, and you can't just will yourself out of it. Although there is a lot you can do for yourself, you may also need professional help.

Typical symptoms of postnatal depression are ongoing, daily and persistent feelings of depression, anxiety, low energy and sadness, with frequent bouts of weeping and crying. Other, additional, symptoms may include:

- Extreme feelings of not being able to cope
- Panic attacks
- Exhaustion and concern about lack of sleep
- Irritability
- Inability to cry despite need
- Feeling out of control
- Inability to concentrate
- Poor memory
- Suicidal thoughts
- Loss of appetite or over-eating
- Sleeping too much
- Insomnia or disturbed sleep (and not just because of your baby)
- Low self-esteem
- Loss of confidence
- Low libido (though this can also be quite normal—see Chapter 6 and 13)
- Lack of interest in life and normal activities
- Difficulty organising normal activities
- Feeling hopeless and helpless
- Feeling trapped/irreversible life sentence
- Fear of being alone
- Fear of social contact
- Increased use of drugs (alcohol, pain killers, cigarettes, etc)
- Denial—fear of admitting to depression because of social stigma, or being labelled a 'bad mother'
- Fear of being a 'bad mother'

This last symptom leads us into another area—your feelings about your baby and motherhood. You may experience excessive anxiety about your baby, and this may be triggered by the guilt you feel over your lack of maternal feelings. You may even have thoughts of hurting your baby and, being fearful of acting out these thoughts, over-compensate by being extra fussy and overly concerned with every real or imagined problem. Alternatively, you might respond with a confused neglect, avoiding contact with your baby so as not to harm him. All of this may lead to feelings of guilt, embarrassment, shame, hopelessness or even anger and resentment.

If your feelings toward your child are still confused, or you haven't yet 'fallen in love', don't panic. The best relationships are often those that mature slowly—just keep caring for your baby and have patience and trust that things will be fine. Every mother has a different experience, even from one birth to the next, and there is no perfect or correct way to be a mother, or feel toward your child. The mystery and inspirations of life come from the huge variety of experiences it offers you—your life and feelings are unique and special, and it would be very tedious if we could all expect the same.

The causes of postnatal depression

The causes of postnatal depression are many. It is the accumulation of the factors unique to each person that lead to 'system overload' and result in the symptoms we have described.

Hormonal changes

The massive drop in oestrogen and progesterone that contributes to the 'Baby Blues' may also be a major cause in postnatal depression, though, as some fathers and adoptive parents experience similar symptoms, there are obviously other contributing factors. Stress and exhaustion, as well as being direct causes of postnatal depression, can also have a negative effect on neuro-hormonal balance, which may not become obvious for several months after the birth.

There are also other hormonal changes that result from pregnancy and birth, and that may be exacerbated by stress or exhaustion, which hinder recovery.

Research conducted in 1995 at the National Institute of Child Health and Human Development in California suggested that there may be irregularities in the production of the stress hormone, cortisol. In a normal stress reaction, the hypothalamus releases a substance that increases the levels of cortisol that helps maintain blood sugar levels and coping mechanisms. During the last three months of pregnancy, this function is taken over by the placenta, probably to help the mother deal with the stress of childbirth. After the birth, when the placenta is expelled, it can take up to 12 weeks for the hypothalamus to resume production. Unfortunately, this is also the time when a woman is experiencing high levels of stress and increased demand on her resources, and this can lead to adrenal exhaustion, especially if the birth was particularly demanding, or involved surgery.

Another theory, the result of research conducted at Edinburgh University, is that the brain level of serotonin is decreased at birth, or that there is a decreased ability to uptake serotonin. This contributes to depression, although the endorphins, dopamine and other neurochemicals that flood the brain at birth, and which give feelings of pleasure and elation, can mask this until some days or weeks after the birth. It can take the body a year or more to return to normal, though under favourable conditions, this will be much sooner rather than later.

Nutritional deficiencies

Both pregnancy and breastfeeding place a high nutritional demand on you, with the foetus receiving first pick of the available nutrients, and this is why we consider preconception and pregnancy nutritional support so important. Indeed we believe this to be the single most important preventative measure that you can take, especially if you believe yourself to be at risk of postnatal depression.

The balance of copper and zinc can be critical at this time, as copper rises during pregnancy to twice its normal level and zinc, to which it is antagonistic, packs into the placenta. When the placenta, which is a storehouse of minerals, is discarded at birth, you lose these minerals (remember that most traditional tribes and animals eat this organ). This can result in a reduction in energy production in every cell in your body which can contribute to postnatal depression, and continuing high copper levels are a further, independent risk factor. If this nutrient imbalance is not addressed, none of the other remedies we suggest will be as effective, and you will be much more susceptible to the effects of hormonal changes.

Other nutritional deficiencies, which can also occur at this time, will increase your risk of postnatal depression. Essential fatty acids (especially the omega 3 variety that are found in fish or flax seeds) are required for healthy brain function and hormonal balance, B-complex vitamins (especially B6 and folic acid) are essential for energy and stress resistance, cholesterol is important for hormone production. All of these may be low after the birth. Iron levels can also become quite depleted during pregnancy, when the volume of your blood increases considerably. Then any blood loss at the birth and the sudden drop in blood volume (30 per cent) can lead to iron deficiency and fatigue.

Emotional, psychological and social factors

There's a huge build-up to the birth of your baby, and you may not have looked beyond this, or you may have simply expected that somehow you would be 'happy ever after' like in those fairy tales you plan to read to your child. Or you may have had unrealistic expectations of how well you would meet the challenges of new motherhood. You may not be used to dealing with someone as unpredictable and demanding as your new baby, especially if he is a 'high needs' baby, and you may have been used to being in control of most aspects of your life. You may need to give up your expectations or your need for control and just 'go with the flow' (turn to Chapter 13 for more on this). You may also need to deal with other people's expectations, pressures to conform to an 'ideal' model of motherhood, or even criticism or unwanted advice.

In fact, it's less important to do it 'right' than to just *be* with your baby, and even if you have little previous experience of infants or children, it shouldn't be hard to learn how to cuddle. The emotions you feel may be intense, and unexpected or unsettling, and you need time to get used to them. Becoming a mother, especially with your first child, is a huge life change, and you may have to give up the previous definitions of yourself which may be central to your self-esteem, and linked to your occupation or activities, from which you now feel isolated.

If you're not getting the sleep or practical help and support you need, this can contribute to depression, and the new demands on your relationship with your partner can undermine the comfort he can offer to you (and you to him). It's not only your adjustment to motherhood that can be difficult, but your joint transformation into parents. Your previous relationship may have been primarily sexual, and now you're feeling too tired, your libido is low, your body image is poor, you may feel fat and not very attractive. Any confusion that you feel may also result from the split in your energy, which is now centred outside of yourself in your child.

You may also be highly conscious of the effect of early childhood experiences on later development, and afraid of the consequences of your actions, or you may be overly compensating for the deficiencies you perceived in your own treatment as an infant. Past difficulties in your own parental and familial relationships can surface at this time. Unmet childhood needs or unresolved childhood traumas can compound your feelings of depression or anxiety, and the feeling that you are the one who needs to be cared for, at the very time when you need to give so much.

It takes time and energy to cope with these emotions, and you may feel that you have none. This can lead to resentment and guilt, which can build to insupportable levels, and lead to neglect of, or over-attention to, your baby. You may need professional help to deal with these issues, especially if they are long-term or have been repressed. Past psychological or psychiatric history may also be a factor, though there are conflicting opinions about this.

Structural changes

During birth, your sacrum can become displaced, and this may affect the proper functioning of the limbic system, which controls emotional aspects of behaviour. Osteopathic treatment of the sacrum and lower back can correct this and may help to resolve symptoms of postnatal depression.

Other risk factors

Some mothers are more likely to be affected by these hormonal, emotional and structural imbalances than others. We've discussed how poor nutrition can increase your risk of suffering from postnatal depression, and other risk factors include:

- Family history of postnatal depression
- Postnatal depression after a previous birth
- Personal history of depression or moodiness (controversial)
- History of severe premenstrual syndrome
- High anxiety through pregnancy
- Low thyroid function
- Low blood sugar
- Early discharge from hospital (some hospitals discharge you after four to eight hours, when you may not be ready or have a satisfactory alternative)
- Alcoholic or dysfunctional family history

- Single or adolescent mother
- Premature, 'compromised' or unusually fussy baby
- Baby with poor nutritional status (will tend to cry more)
- Lack of financial support
- Lack of self-care (diet, exercise, interest in life)
- Traumatic birth (e.g. Caesarean)
- Use of mini-pill (leads to nutritional deficiencies)

Overcoming postnatal depression

Many of the things you can do are obvious once you've understood the risk factors. They include:

- Get enough sleep/rest/relaxation

- Get some time to yourself

- Do things you enjoy

- Have company (though not too much)

- Eat well (especially protein-providing foods)

- Take comprehensive nutritional supplements

- Drink plenty of purified water

- Have your iron levels checked (a simple blood test)

- Keep your sense of humour

- Don't try to be superwoman

- Get help with the housework

- Don't do the housework

- Try yoga/tai chi/meditation

- Have a massage

- Avoid alcohol (it's a depressant)

- Avoid sugar (it'll increase blood sugar imbalance)

- Exercise regularly (30 minutes a day)

- Get out of doors

- Breastfeed on demand (helps to moderate hormonal swings, increase endorphins, helps bonding)

- Keep your baby in your bed (more bonding, less exhausting)

- Feel safe about expressing 'unacceptable' feelings about your baby

- Join a 'new mothers' group

- Eat the placenta (rich in minerals; you can cook it like liver)

- Seek advice from the professionals. These include your naturopath, acupuncturist, homoeopath, herbalist, masseur, midwife, osteopath, early childhood nurse, baby clinic sister, GP, local community counselling service and other support groups and institutions (see Contacts and Resources).

Nurturing nutrients

You have an increased need at this time for zinc, calcium, magnesium, vitamin C, B-complex vitamins, the essential fatty acids and possibly iron. As iron competes with zinc, you should establish need (through a blood test) before taking supplements, which should always be organic. Eat and supplement as we suggest in Chapter 4.

Healing herbs

Herbal remedies can calm you down (nervines), help you deal with stress (adaptogens) and balance your hormones and your endocrine function. Here are some suggestions, though your herbalist will be able to help you choose more effectively.

Nervines

Lemon Balm (specific for melancholy but not if your thyroid is under-active), Lavender (also for guilt and shame), Rosemary (also helps cerebral function), Vervain (also convalescent), Valerian (especially if anxious), Skullcap (especially in hyper-adrenal states), Passiflora (for depression with 'spiritual torment'), St John's Wort (shown in clinical trials to help depression), Oats (a good nerve tonic), Zizyphus, Chamomile (both good for insomnia), Kava (especially for anxiety), Piscidia (for sleep problems and pain), Pulsatilla (especially for changeable moods), *Damiana* (anti-depressive), and *Motherwort* (also a good hormone tonic).

Adaptogens
Withania, *Siberian* and *Korean Ginseng*, *Astragalus*, *Rehmannia*, *Schisandra*, *Gotu Kola* and *Liquorice* (also a good hormonal tonic).

Hormonal balancers
False Unicorn Root, *Peony*, *Chastetree* (also good for milk production), *Ladies Mantle*, *Raspberry*, *Dong Quai*, *Blue Cohosh*, *Sarsparilla* and *Saw Palmetto*.

Herbs for brain function
Ginkgo and *Rosemary*.

Nutritive herbs
Nettles, *Alfalfa*, *Fennel* and *Fenugreek* (all of these also help lactation).

Bitter herbs
St Mary's Thistle, *Dandelion* and *Blessed Thistle* (all bitter herbs can help depressive states).

These herbs can be taken as teas, or prescribed as herbal extracts by your medical herbalist. Although any herbal (or other) remedies you take will be transmitted to your baby through the breast milk, this will be to a very limited extent and should not cause any harm. However, if your baby seems upset or disturbed, you should stop the remedy (and see if he improves).

Helpful homoeopathics
Here are a few homoeopathic remedies which are specific for postnatal depression:

- *Aconite* (if fearful)

- *Apis* (for constant weeping)

- *Arsenicum album* (if restless at night and fearful or suicidal)

- *Aurum metallicum* (if feeling unworthy or quarrelsome)

- *China* (if exhausted after blood loss)
- *Ignatia* (for sadness, sensitivity, moodiness, changeable emotions)
- *Lilium tigrinum* (for profound depression)
- *Lycopodium* (if melancholic or afraid to be alone)
- *Nat Mur* (if moody and depressed)
- *Phosphorus* (if you need sympathy, touch or are very fearful)
- *Pulsatilla* (if moody, tearful and restless)
- *Sepia* (for feelings of indifference towards your baby and fear of real and imaginary things)
- *Silica* (for dread of failure)

Favourable flower essences

The flower essence remedies that you may find especially helpful at this time include:

- *Aspen* (for vague fears)
- *Cherry Plum* (for fear of losing control and reason)
- *Clematis* (for lack of interest)
- *Crab Apple* (for poor body image)
- *Gentian* (for discouragement)
- *Gorse* (for hopelessness and despair)
- *Mimulus* (for specific fears)
- *Mustard* (for deep melancholy)
- *Olive* (for exhaustion)
- *Pine* (for guilt)
- *Red Chestnut* (for fear for others)
- *Scleranthus* (for changing moods)
- *Star of Bethlehem* (for delayed shock)
- *Sweet Chestnut* (for extreme anguish)

⚘ *Walnut* (for protection against outside influence and major life changes)

⚘ *White Chestnut* (for unwanted thoughts)

⚘ *Wild Oat* (for uncertainty regarding life's path)

Effective essential oils

These can be used in a burner, a compress or as part of massage. Particularly helpful at this time are:

⚘ *Clary Sage* (sedative but also vitalising)

⚘ *Geranium* (for hormone balance and anxiety)

⚘ *Jasmine* (uplifting and soothing)

⚘ *Lavender* (for depression and stress)

⚘ *Melissa* (uplifting)

⚘ *Neroli* (calming and uplifting)

⚘ *Rose* (if you feel vulnerable or sad)

⚘ *Ylang Ylang* (sedating)

Relaxing reflexology

The areas on the feet that can be massaged to help at this time are those that affect the endocrine system, solar plexus, uterus and ovaries (see diagram). Massage of the second toe can help you to feel more centred and settled in yourself.

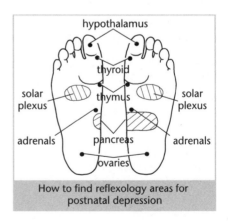

How to find reflexology areas for postnatal depression

Marvellous massage

It's not just your feet that need attention—you could do with an all-over rub. You can ask the masseuse to use the essential oils we've suggested, and play relaxing music. Everyone deserves this treat.

Comforting counselling, therapy and support groups

There are support groups for sufferers of postnatal depression which offer counselling (see Contacts and Resources) or you may prefer a personal recommendation. Hypnotherapy can also be extremely effective (see Chapter 7 for more on this).

Medical support

If you feel that, despite our suggestions, you are not responding well, you should seek medical help. This will usually include many aspects of what we have discussed so far, with counselling and emotional support in both one-to-one and group situations. Antidepressants are occasionally prescribed, though studies have shown adverse effects in some breastfed infants. Some antidepressants are more of a potential problem than others. Prozac, for example, can cross the barrier into the breast milk, and tricyclic antidepressants, such as Tryptanol, can cause withdrawal problems for your baby. If all else fails, and you resort to drug therapy, make sure you and your doctor seek out a medicine that doesn't cross over into the breast milk. On the very rare occasions when hospitalisation is required, it is common practice not to separate mother and baby.

While the causes of postnatal depression are complex, we feel there's little doubt that the high (and increasing) incidence of this condition is closely linked to modern diets and lifestyles, and to present birthing practices. If you follow our recommendations before conception and during pregnancy, and if you have a natural, unmedicated birth, you'll have the best possible chance of thoroughly enjoying the early months (and years) with your new baby as nature clearly intended them to be enjoyed!

Care after birth for you and your baby

Even if your labour was over in a flash and you feel 'ready to run a marathon', don't even think about it! Even if you're not suffering from exhaustion or shock, you'll still need some postpartum care after being the star of the show. (Your baby might too—more of that later.) You could have a herbal formulation ready for use at this time, which could include:

- *False Unicorn Root* and *Blue Cohosh* (as uterine tonics).
- *Nettle* (for essential nutrients, and to stabilise your blood sugar levels).
- *Calendula* (to prevent infection and promote healing).
- *Shepherd's Purse* (for any bleeding).
- *Lavender* (for calming and healing).
- *Uva Ursi* (to prevent urinary tract infections).

If you are exhausted, herbs such as *Dong Quai*, *Withania*, *Ginger*, *Liquorice* and *Ginseng* could be added to this mix, and you may benefit from the Bach Flower remedy *Olive*. The homoeopathic remedy for this time is *Secale cornutum*, especially if you're feeling hot. If you've lost a lot of blood, your midwife should check to see whether you're anaemic.

For shock, you can use *Motherwort*, *Rescue Remedy* and homoeopathic *Arnica*, at the '30c' potency, three times daily for three days.

PERINEAL CARE

The pelvic floor exercises, massage (external only) and essential oils that we suggested in Chapter 5 for preparation of your perineum can also aid recovery from any damage to this area that occurred during the birth. You can use *Arnica* or *Witch Hazel* ointment for any bruising (though not on broken skin) and ice packs if there is swelling (these work best during the first 24 hours). You can try sitz-baths with essential oils such as *Lavender* or the herbs *Calendula* and *Comfrey*, or use the herbs to make poultices or compresses. *St John's Wort* (*Hypericum*) oil is particularly helpful to heal any damaged nerve endings (see Chapter 5 for how to prepare this oil) and massage of the reflex zone for the perineum can also assist recovery (see diagrams page 279).

If you've been cut or have torn during the birth, you will probably need to lie on your stomach or side as often as possible, instead of sitting. You will also need to hold the stitched areas firmly with a clean sanitary pad when you're having a bowel motion and, since urine will burn the raw wound, you should try pouring water over the perineal area as you urinate. You can use any squirting type bottle for this, with *Calendula* or *Golden Seal* added to the water.

Other herbs to consider for ointments, creams, poultices, compresses or sitz-baths are *Aloe Vera*, *Yarrow*, *Chamomile*, *Sage*, *Rosemary* and *Myrrh*. These aid healing and prevent infection. Additional essential oils for bathing or massaging are *Cypress*, which is astringent and will help the wound to heal, *Lemon* and *Bergamot*, which are both antiseptic. Creams and ointments should not be applied until the wound is dry and closed, when they can assist the later stages of healing and prevent scar tissue from forming, but sitz-baths and poultices can be used two to three times a day directly after the birth. Be careful, when massaging, not to stretch the area if you have stitches. *Gotu Kola* is a very effective herb to use when a wound is healing, and appropriate homoeopathic remedies include:

- *Arnica* (if the stitches are painful or there is a lot of bruising).
- *Calendula* (if there is infection).
- *Hypericum* (if the wound is slow to heal).
- *Staphysagria* (to help heal any incision or wound).

RECOVERY AFTER A CAESAREAN SECTION OR EPIDURAL

Any of the remedies recommended above for wound healing or infection apply equally to recovery from a Caesarean or an episiotomy. However, with a Caesarean (or epidural), there is the added problem of the effects of anaesthesia. Studies show that the risk of headache and backache is increased after an epidural, but osteopathy can prevent and treat both problems.

Recovery from the effects of an anaesthetic is faster and more complete if you use detoxifying liver remedies such as *Dandelion Root*, *Schisandra* or *St Mary's Thistle*. The homoeopathic remedy for recovery is *Thuja*, with *Hypericum* for nerve damage if you had an epidural, and *Ginger* tea if you are feeling nauseated. If you're suffering from intestinal gas, bring your knees to your chest and hold them there by wrapping your arms around them, and the gas will release. If the anaesthesia was administered through your respiratory system, practise deep breathing as recommended for relaxation in Chapter 7. The reflexology zones needing attention are those for the uterus, the spine (if you had an epidural), the lungs and chest (if you had a general anaesthetic), the colon (if you have a problem with gas) and the liver (for detoxification). See the diagrams in Appendix 1, page 279 to locate these zones.

URINARY TRACT INFECTION

Urination can sometimes be difficult directly after the birth, especially in the first 24 hours, since your bladder suddenly has more room to expand. It may also have been traumatised or bruised during delivery and become temporarily paralysed, or it may be less sensitive due to the drugs or anaesthetic that were administered. There may be reflex spasms in the urethra from any perineal pain, you may also be fearful of experiencing pain when you urinate, or, if you've had surgery, embarrassed at having to use a bed pan.

You should empty your bladder within six to eight hours after the birth, as failure to do so could lead to a urinary tract infection, loss of muscle tone and possibly bleeding if the expanded bladder hinders the normal descent of the womb.

If the urine just won't flow, here are some things that will help:

- Drink lots of purified water.

- Take a walk.

- Turn on the tap and listen to the running water.

- Whistle.

- Pour water over your urethral opening (or use a peri-bottle).

- Apply warmth (sitz-bath) or cold (ice packs).

- Use diuretic herbs (such as *Dandelion Leaf, Couch Grass* and *Cleavers,* or *Buchu, Parsley, Corn Silk* and *Wild Carrot* (these last four are not for use during pregnancy).

- Massage the reflex zones for the kidneys, ureters and bladder. (See the diagrams in Appendix 1, page 279.)

- Use the homoeopathic remedies *Aconitum, Arsenicum album* and *Causticum.*

To prevent or treat urinary tract infection, you should:

- Do all of the above.

- Wipe front to back.

- Wear loose cotton underwear.

- Avoid bath preparations (except essential oils such as *Sandalwood, Lavender* or *Bergamot*).

- Stay away from coffee, tea, alcohol, soft drinks, nicotine, sugar and spicy foods (we know, we know—you weren't even tempted!).

- Eat well (don't fast).

- Eat 'live' yoghurt, parsley and garlic.

- Increase your intake of vitamins A, B-complex, C (with bioflavonoids) and E, and zinc.

- Add freshly squeezed lemon juice to your water.

- Drink unsweetened *Cranberry* juice (one glass every hour for up to 10 hours).

- Use demulcent herbs (those soothing to the mucous membranes) such as *Cleavers*, *Marshmallow*, *Corn Silk*, *Liquorice*, *Couch Grass* and *Horsetail* (not in pregnancy).

- Use urinary antiseptic herbs such as *Buchu*, *Uva Ursi* (not in pregnancy), *Thyme*, *Echinacea* and *Garlic*.

- Treat your kidneys with *Nettle* and *Cleavers* (if they are painful, seek medical attention).

- Try not to use antibiotics (but don't let any infection go untreated).

- Drink *Barley* water. Add half a cup of barley to three litres of boiling water. Simmer for 20 minutes, cool and strain. Add the juice of a freshly squeezed lemon and drink throughout the day.

CONSTIPATION

It's not only urination that might be difficult after giving birth; your bowels may also seize up. There are several reasons for this. Your bowel may have been completely emptied during labour and you may not have eaten since. Your bowel, like your bladder, may have been traumatised or bruised and the muscles in your abdomen may have been thoroughly stretched and weakened. You may also be afraid of pain in the perineal area, or of bursting your stitches. Here's what you can do to get things moving happily again.

- Drink plenty of purified water.

- Add the freshly squeezed juice of a lemon to warm water and drink first thing in the morning.

- Eat plenty of roughage (fresh fruit and vegetables).

❋ Move around.

❋ Take *Acidophilus* and *Slippery Elm* powder.

❋ Use bulking agents such as *Psyllium*.

❋ Avoid laxatives if possible, but if you need them use gentle herbs such as *Dandelion Root*.

❋ Stimulate the reflex zones for the colon (large intestine) and rectum. (See the diagrams in Appendix 1, page 279.)

❋ Practice your pelvic floor exercises.

❋ Use massage in a clockwise direction over the abdomen (you can add essential oils such as *Mandarin* or *Orange*), or up the stomach meridian which runs along the outside of the thigh from the hip to just below the knee to keep the bowels regular. You can also try reflexology for the colon, massaging the foot arches in a clockwise direction, a massage of the lower back with relaxing essential oils such as *Lavender* or *Bergamot*, or osteopathy (for practitioner referrals, see Contacts and Resources).

❋ Try homoeopathic remedies such as *Nux vomica*, *Nat mur*, *Bryonia* and *Sepia*. As we've mentioned before, the correct choice of homoeopathic remedy is usually best left to a qualified practitioner.

❋ Try acupressure on the following points:

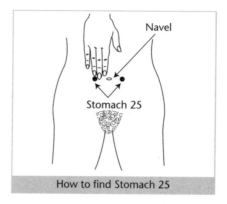

How to find Stomach 25

Stomach 25: two finger widths on either side of your belly button (the third finger will find the spot). Use dispersing action on this point.

Colon 4: in the apex of the 'V' shape formed by the bones of the index finger and the thumb, on the back of your hand. Use dispersing action but, as this point is often very sore, increase the pressure slowly. *This point must not be used in pregnancy.*

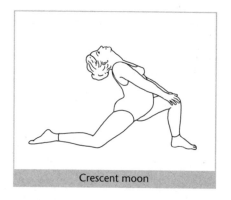
Crescent moon

Triple Heater 6: this point is on the outer side of the forearm, between the two bones, at four fingers' distance from the bend of the wrist. Use dispersing action. *This point should be used with caution in the sixth month of pregnancy.*

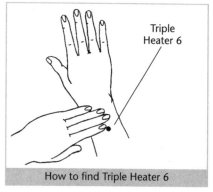
Triple Heater 6

How to find Triple Heater 6

AFTER-PAINS AND SUBINVOLUTION

As your uterus returns to its pre-pregnancy size, you may experience some cramping pains. These are not usually too bad with your first baby, since your uterus recovers more easily. This will also be the case if you've followed our recommendations for preconception and pregnancy health care and have good nutritional status. However, in some cases, the pains can continue for several days, and can be quite strong, especially during breastfeeding, which stimulates the uterus to contract. If the pains are really severe, talk to your midwife or other carer, as there may be clots or retained tissue causing the problem. Here are some suggestions for helping your uterus return quickly and painlessly to its normal size.

⚕ Breastfeed on demand.

⚕ Use essential oils of *Chamomile, Lavender* and *Marjoram* in your bath or to massage your belly.

- Get plenty of calcium and magnesium (try the tissue salts).

- Helpful herbs include *Blue* and *Black Cohosh*, *Cramp Bark*, *Black Haw*, *Raspberry*, *Motherwort* and *St John's Wort*.

- Homoeopathic remedies to choose from are *Belladonna*, *Calc carb*, *Caulophyllum*, *Chamomilla*, *Cimicifuga*, *Pulsatilla*, *Sabina*, *Sepia* and *Sulphur*. If you can't consult a homoeopath to choose the right remedy, check the indications we've given earlier.

- Take homoeopathic *Arnica* before and after giving birth to prevent bruising and trauma.

- Try massaging the reflex zones for the uterus. (See the diagrams in Appendix 1, page 279.)

VULVAL HAEMATOMA

Some women suffer from this condition after giving birth as a result of a rupture of a vulval varicose vein. If there's excessive blood loss or swelling (it can reach the size of a pear) you should seek medical help.

If you've been assiduous with your intake of nutrients, especially vitamin C and the bioflavonoids and *Nettle* tea, you are unlikely to have this problem. However, if you do, you can try *Tienchi Ginseng*, 1 mL of the fluid extract every two hours, *Witch Hazel* and *Horsechestnut* with vitamin E cream applied to the affected area.

PREPARATION FOR BREASTFEEDING

As the title of our next book is *The Natural Way to Better Breastfeeding*, we won't extend this already over-long volume (in our editors' opinions, anyway!) by telling you everything you need to know about this topic. However, we can't resist giving you a few hints to get you started. Early and correct establishment of breastfeeding is vital and one of the most important factors in ensuring that you'll be able to breastfeed successfully for as long as your baby needs to.

Breast milk is what your baby needs to thrive, and breastfeeding is an important part of the bonding process. It's also infinitely easier for you than all the fuss and bother of bottle sterilisation and formula preparation. We could wax on for pages, but we'll (and you'll) have to wait! Here are a few essential pointers for getting started:

- Relax and get enough sleep (with your baby sleeping beside you is the only way to achieve this).

- Drink plenty of purified water and fluids (not cow's milk).

- Feed on demand. Let your baby suckle as often and for as long as possible. Remember he's getting comfort as well as nutrition at your breast.

- Keep your baby in your bed so he can suck intermittently all night (and you don't have to get out of bed).

- Don't give your baby (and don't let him be given) any supplementary formula or sugar water.

- Eat plenty of nutritious foods: especially helpful are grains (particularly barley, oats and brown rice), leafy greens, red and orange vegetables, avocadoes, nuts (especially almonds) and seaweed (make sure they're organic).

- Try juicing your vegetables: the nutrients are more readily available and you'll get more of them.

- Add lots of garlic to your food—most babies like it, and two clinical trials have shown benefit. However, some babies get irritated by it and get loose stools.

- Keep taking your nutritional supplements.

- Drink teas made from *Nettle, Alfalfa, Fenugreek, Fennel, Dandelion, Chamomile* and *Raspberry*.

- Use the culinary herbs and spices *Coriander, Cumin, Caraway, Dill* and *Aniseed* in your cooking.

- Use the herbs *St Mary's Thistle, Chastetree, Vervain, Goat's Rue, Catnip, Cleavers, Blessed Thistle, Marshmallow* and *Squaw Vine*.

- Avoid *Parsley* and *Sage* in large quantities, unless you have too much milk, since they will dry it up. (Give any excess to a milk bank for premature babies instead—if you can find one—or you can freeze it if you want to go out without your baby once in a while.)

⚘ Beer (or guinness/stout) has been used as a traditional remedy to increase breast milk, but since we don't recommend alcohol when you're breastfeeding you can try *Hops*. This is what beer is made from and the reason that it's a useful remedy.

⚘ Get yourself a good, comfortable nursing bra or three (see Contacts and Resources).

⚘ Try stimulating Gall Bladder 21, using tonifying pressure. To find this point, draw a straight line up from the nipple. This point is where it crosses the top of the shoulder.

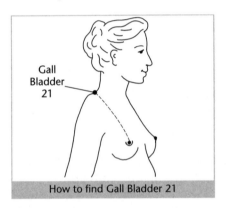

How to find Gall Bladder 21

⚘ Massage the reflex zones for the breasts. (See the diagrams in Appendix 1, page 279.)

⚘ Gently massage your breasts, with the palm of your hands, in a clockwise direction.

⚘ Try the homoeopathic remedies *Calc carb* (if you have a lot of milk, but your baby is reluctant to feed—remember, breast milk looks watery in comparison to cow's milk), *Pulsatilla* (if there's poor supply due to stress and anxiety) or *Lac defloratum* (if your milk dries up altogether).

SORE OR INFECTED BREASTS

If your breasts get congested, engorged or infected or your nipples feel sore, there are a number of remedies you can try. You should also encourage your baby to nurse as much as possible on the affected side, as sometimes the problem simply lies with the ducts becoming kinked, and feeding will help to unblock them.

- Apply a poultice, compress or ointment of *Poke Root*, *Comfrey*, *Parsley*, *Marshmallow Root* or essential oils *Geranium*, *Rose* and *Lavender*. Use only tepid water in the compress or poultice, since your breasts will usually be hot.

- Put bruised or steamed *Cabbage* or *Comfrey* leaves in your bra, or a poultice of raw, mashed potato (very tasty! and sexy to boot!).

- Massage the reflex zones for the breasts and the axillary lymphatics. (See the diagrams in Appendix 1, page 279.)

- If your breasts are swollen and lumpy, with pain radiating all over your body, take the homoeopathic version of *Poke Root* internally. This remedy is called *Phytolacca*. (*Poke Root* is too toxic to take as a herb when you're breastfeeding.)

- Other helpful homoeopathic remedies are *Belladonna* (for too much milk with breasts that are hot, swollen, rock hard and tender to touch), *Bryonia* (if your breasts are hot and painful), or *Sulphur* (if there is infection or if your nipples smart and burn after feeding).

- For sore or cracked nipples, try *Chamomilla* (for inflamed and very tender nipples), *Lycopodium* (for cracked nipples that bleed during feeds), *Staphysagria* (for extreme nipple pain when feeding).

- *Garlic*, *Propolis*, *Echinacea*, *Golden Seal*, *Myrrh* and vitamin C are helpful if there's an infection. If your baby gets diarrhoea, you may need to reduce the dose of vitamin C.

- *Calendula* cream can soften and soothe sensitive nipples (make sure to wash it off carefully before a feed).

- *Lavender* and *Rose* essential oils can soothe sore nipples. Use a very dilute mixture of one drop in a teaspoon of nut oil and massage directly into your nipples after each feed. Remember to wash the whole areola and nipple thoroughly before the next feed.

Candida infection is another possible reason for painful breasts. You will be alerted to this possibility by the presence of thrush (white, curdy coating) in your baby's mouth. Treatment includes dietary control (no sugars or refined carbohydrates), gut recolonisation with lactobacilli and the use of fungicidal remedies. For more details see our previous books *The Natural Way to Better Babies* and *The Natural Way to a Better Pregnancy*. Your baby may need treatment too.

NATURAL CONTRACEPTION

We know that having another baby is the last thing on your mind, and even sex may not be high on your list of priorities right now. If you are fully breastfeeding (as we hope you are), it's unlikely that you'll be fertile for a while, as Mother Nature ensures good spacing between conceptions, allowing you time to recover and restore adequate nutritional status so your next conception, pregnancy and baby are as healthy as possible.

However, you can't rely on this process, and conceptions have been known to occur within two weeks of birth, even in women who are fully breastfeeding. So it's wise to consider what contraception you would prefer to use, right away. We'll cover this subject more fully in our next book, *The Natural Way to Better Breastfeeding*, but just want to put in a word of warning here.

The mini-pill, which is usually prescribed for lactating mothers, has significant deleterious effects on your nutritional status, and therefore on what you provide for your baby, as well as possible hormonal effects. The health concerns for users of the oral contraceptive pill are also considerable (see our previous books *The Natural Way to Better Babies* and *Natural Fertlity*).

One alternative is to use condoms, but you can improve the situation, and reduce the occasions when this is necessary, by monitoring your fertility and knowing when you are at risk (which may not be for several months). For more on natural methods of birth control see Contacts and Resources where you can find details of natural contraception kits available through Francesca's company *Natural Fertility Management*, and her book *Natural Fertility*.

HOMOEOPATHIC REMEDIES FOR AN ENDANGERED, SHOCKED OR BRUISED BABY

Just like you, even a baby who's been through a better birth may need some care. Of course, if your baby is in danger, and his vital signs are weak, medical attention is required immediately. However, there have been some remarkable recoveries attributed to homoeopathic remedies. These are easy to administer to a newborn baby, entirely non-toxic, and cannot interfere with any necessary medical treatment. A few drops under your baby's tongue cannot be contraindicated in any way, and may make an important contribution to his recovery. The first and almost universally applicable remedy is 'Rescue Remedy', a combination of Bach Flower essences. If you want to have some of this on hand, you may prefer to have a small bottle made up in a base of distilled water. The usual base of one-third brandy and two-thirds water may not be appropriate for a newborn baby, even though the few drops given will contain minimal alcohol. If you use a plain water base, the remedy should be kept in the fridge, but not for longer than two weeks, since there is no alcohol present to act as a preservative.

Other homoeopathic remedies which could be appropriate are:

- *Aconitum:* if your baby is shrieking in terror or panic, if he is purple and breathless.

- *Arnica:* if your baby is suffering from severe bruising, cranial haemorrhage or other bleeding, shock or trauma.

- *Belladonna:* if your baby's face is flushed, and his pupils dilated.

- *Carbo vegetabilis:* if your baby is limp, flaccid, blue, grey, cold, collapsed, or close to death.

- *Laurocerasus:* if your baby is blue, gasping for air and breath, and lacking in reaction, or does not breathe after mucus suction.

If you need to administer homoeopathic or any other natural medicine to your baby, but cannot get him to accept it, the alternative route is via your breast milk. Though some substances don't pass the breast barrier very efficiently, a more substantial dose taken by you is likely to filter down, in suitably smaller doses, to your child.

If your baby has been bruised during the birth, use *Arnica* internally, as suggested above, and also use an *Arnica* or *Hypericum* (*St John's Wort*) oil, lotion or cream. These should be made from the actual plant (not the homoeopathic extract), should be pure, and contain no other ingredients or additives. Some of the proprietary brands available in health food or chemist shops might contain other herbs that could be too abrasive for your baby's skin. *Arnica* ointment should not be used on broken skin.

NEONATAL JAUNDICE

Jaundice is a common problem with newborn babies. It can vary from a mild condition that can benefit from the remedies we describe below, to a severe condition requiring medical attention. The yellow skin and eyes that are typical of a jaundiced baby are due to the presence of a substance called *bilirubin*. This is a yellow coloured by-product of the process whereby your baby gets rid of excess red blood cells. In utero, in order to get oxygen from the blood that is filtered through the placenta, your baby needs more red blood cells than he requires once he's breathing independently.

Physiological jaundice

When jaundice is simply the result of a normal process, it's called 'physiological' jaundice. It usually appears about three days after the birth, peaks the next day, and is gone two days later. As long as your baby seems otherwise healthy, alert and happy, you need not be concerned. In fact, there is considerable opinion that this form of jaundice is protective and of benefit. If your baby does not seem well, if he has poor muscle tone, is lethargic and sleeping excessively, isn't feeding well or is vomiting, and is generally querulous and unhappy, he will need medical attention. Bilirubin levels that are too high for him to eliminate can lead to severe ill-effects, including brain damage.

Your baby is at greater risk of dangerous levels of bilirubin if he is premature, if you have not been healthy during your pregnancy, and especially if medication or trauma accompanied the birth. Similarly, any medication that you take while breastfeeding (such as the mini-pill) can create a greater risk for your child. To prevent jaundice reaching dangerous levels, here are some preventative measures that you can take.

- Follow our recommendations for the preconception period and pregnancy—this means good nutrition, healthy lifestyle and avoiding toxins.

- Avoid medication; take active steps to experience a natural birth.

- Avoid vitamin K injections for your baby; these increase the risk of jaundice.

- Drink plenty of herbal teas in later pregnancy, especially those which promote healthy liver function (*Dandelion Root*) and provide vitamin K (*Nettle, Alfalfa*).

- Breastfeed on demand from birth onwards.

- Leave the cord intact; cut it only when it has stopped pulsating.

- Make sure your baby receives plenty of natural sunlight in the early morning and late afternoon.

If you need to treat your baby for jaundice, here's what to do.

- Take liver herbs yourself (*Dandelion Root, St Mary's Thistle* or *Schisandra*) as teas or fluid extracts. Your baby will get his dose through your breast milk.

- In severe cases, and with professional supervision, these herbs can be given directly to your baby. Place a few drops under his tongue, every four hours, or rub a few drops on your nipple before feeds. Alternatively, there are remedies called 'Homoeobotanicals'. These are herbs, potentised like a homoeopathic remedy, that can be given in very small doses. This treatment should only be continued for a few days, or until the condition improves.

- Put a few drops of the homoeopathic remedy *Aconite* (in '200c' potency) on your nipples before each feed. This should only be done for a single day.

- Place one red and one blue veil over your baby's sleeping place, to filter the sunlight and create a violet light. This is a low-tech alternative to the ultra-violet lamps that are used in medical or hospital situations. It avoids the problem of electro-magnetic fields surrounding your child.

✳ Keep breastfeeding, even if you are still only producing colostrum. Use the remedies suggested previously if your milk supply diminishes.

Breast milk jaundice

Breastfed babies can experience jaundice as a result of hormones that come through the milk. This form of the condition appears a bit later, any time from the fifth day after the birth to two weeks later, and can last several weeks. Again, if your baby seems happy, alert and healthy, there is no need to be concerned.

For treatment, similar measures to those described above should be sufficient. However, you may be advised to stop breastfeeding if the condition is resulting in particularly high levels of bilirubin. If so, seek advice from the Nursing Mothers Association for a second opinion and advice on how to handle the situation. Any break in feeding should be seen as a last resort, and only contemplated if your baby is obviously sick and not responding to other measures. If you do need to wean your baby temporarily, be sure to keep expressing your milk so that your supply doesn't diminish. Use goat's milk (with *Acidophilus* added) for your baby, and don't stop breastfeeding for more than one or two days at most. Fortunately, it's usually possible to avoid this drastic measure.

Pathological jaundice

If jaundice appears directly after the birth, or within the first two days, it may be due to some infection or liver condition. Though you can use all the remedies we've suggested here, you should also seek medical attention.

CARE OF WOUNDS

One wound that all babies will have after birth is at the navel where the umbilical cord was cut. Another might be on your baby boy's penis where he was circumcised (although we certainly hope that our words on this subject in Chapter 10 will deter you from this mutilation). Keeping a wound clean and free from infection is important, and usually simple. You should keep the stump of the cord warm and dry, and fasten nappies so they don't rub it. The stump should take between five and ten days to dry up completely and fall off. Usually, all you need to do is to keep it clean. Use some soft cotton material (this is preferable to a cotton swab or cotton wool, which may leave wisps behind) dipped in rubbing (or surgical) alcohol or *Witch Hazel* (a more pleasant alternative). If there is a bad smell or inflammation and you suspect infection, saline (antiseptic), or an infusion of *Rosemary* (antiseptic and astringent) or *Calendula* flowers (also anti-microbial) could be used. Breast milk is often recommended, as it is full of antibodies that fight infection, and the appropriate herbs are *Myrrh* (usually used as a powder), *Golden Seal* and *Echinacea*. You can also take these internally and they'll pass through the breast milk. Occasionally, if required, the herb itself or the homoeobotanical remedies can be given directly to your baby (with supervision from a herbalist). *Propolis* is another useful anti-infective agent.

If healing is slow, *Comfrey* or *Mugwort* leaves can be crushed, put inside a *Cabbage* leaf and used as a poultice. *Arnica* can be applied to reduce bruising, though it should not be used on broken skin, and *St John's Wort* (oil, fluid extract or ointment) can promote the healing of nerve endings.

CRANIAL MISALIGNMENT

During childbirth, the pressure experienced in the birth canal can cause the bones in your baby's head to become misaligned, leading to various problems. Your baby may be jumpy and irritable, suffer from ailments such as colic and sticky eye, cry excessively or have problems sleeping and feeding. The condition may be worse if the birth was traumatic or difficult.

Osteopaths who specialise in cranio-sacral adjustments work extremely gently to correct subtle fluctuations of cerebro-spinal fluid and cranial bone alignment. The results can be spectacular and can correct all the symptoms described above, and many others. However, it's important, for best results, to have your baby treated before the bones of his skull finally set in place.

BRAIN HEMISPHERE IMBALANCE

Kinesiology uses touch along the acupuncture meridians and at pressure points to gently re-balance energy patterns in the body, and is particularly helpful in correcting the left and right brain hemisphere imbalance which is a common problem resulting from a difficult birth. An imbalance that is not corrected can manifest later in life as dyslexia, clumsiness, poor hand-eye coordination, left-handedness, lack of handedness, and visual problems. Early correction is very helpful for these and other subtle effects of birth trauma.

BABY MASSAGE

Your baby is just like you. He loves to be massaged. Most mothers (and fathers) do this instinctively, though some new parents are afraid they may hurt their babies. Baby massage is actually a very old art that is making a come-back. It may now be practised by a trained masseur, is taught to new and prospective parents, and has been introduced into quite a few hospitals, especially in the intensive care units. There are special classes, if you feel you need instruction (see Contacts and Resources), or you can just follow your intuition. Nut oils are a good choice for your baby's skin, but avoid so-called 'baby' oils because they have a petrochemical base.

Of course, you also deserve a massage—and many other treats! We hope that the remedies for you and your newborn baby are just part of a comprehensive program of support for you both, as you both deserve to be cherished and fussed over after your star performances. One thing you both certainly need is plenty of rest, and the chance to have a full and rewarding bonding experience, as we'll explore in the next chapter.

Bonding with your baby

Bonding is all about falling in love with your baby! Nature has perfected an extraordinarily effective scheme to ensure that your child will be loved, cared for, protected and nurtured. The bond formed between the two of you is the means by which nature provides for your infant's physical and emotional wellbeing. The bond also has a direct bearing on how you relate and respond to your baby.

So that you really understand what 'better' bonding means, and how it can take place to best advantage, we're going to describe the ways in which traditional societies treat their newborn babies.

TRADITIONAL NURTURING

As we saw in Chapter 1, in traditional communities, birth usually occurs amongst other women: family members, close friends and a traditional birth attendant such as a midwife or doula. These women are there to give comfort and emotional support. They will also physically support the mother as she labours, they will prepare food and drink for her, they will take care of her older children and will invariably participate in some sort of celebration when the baby is born. The infant is born into warm welcoming arms and he remains there for the first months of his life.

The covering of vernix, which protects and insulates the baby's skin in utero, may still cover his body at birth, and will rub into his skin during the following days or at his first massage. There are very few places in the world where a new baby is not massaged regularly during the first few months or years of his life. Different communities concentrate on massaging different areas—in India and Hawaii, emphasis is placed on massaging the face since it is thought that makes the baby more beautiful. The Maori massage the baby's ankles and knees so he will be graceful and supple. Whatever the reason for massage, the routine is usually carried out using a warm nut or vegetable oil and is always performed in the community's traditional way. The new mother has watched other women perform the massage and she now conveys her love to her new baby through the language that he understands best—the language of touch.

Because the baby is not dirty, his first bath may take place hours, or even days after his birth, and provides an environment that is just as relaxing as the watery one he recently left. This bath is, and has been, valued as part of the bonding process in cultures all over the world from ancient times. The ancient Spartans used myrtle and wine in their infant's first bath and in medieval times soothing herbs such as chamomile, lavender or rose petals were added to the water. In the present day, the custom remains in most indigenous cultures. The Mbuti of Zaire use the water yielded by a huge vine in the forest, to bond the infant to the forest from which he is believed to come. The Ingalik melt ice for their baby's first bath, consuming precious firewood in the process, and thereafter they simply lick their baby's hands and face clean. Indeed, the tradition in eighteenth-century Europe was to lick the child all over. A soothing massage and an equally soothing bath means that the newborn is completely at ease and relaxed.

In the early weeks following the birth the new mother is cared for and cosseted. She is given special food and drink, and spends the time resting. In Japan, the new mother's feet never touch the floor for 40 days, Muslim women are supported for a similar period and Australian Aboriginal mothers enjoy special care for three months after the birth. This period of recuperation and adjustment allows the new mother to regain her strength, and to really get to know her new baby, who never leaves her arms. The baby's introduction to the goings-on in his new environment is quite slow and gradual, for his mother usually spends the early weeks of his life quietly, in her own home.

However as soon as she takes up her normal routine and her place in society again, her baby is firmly attached to her body in some form of sling, and he accompanies her wherever she goes and is part of whatever activity she undertakes. The woman finds it completely unthinkable to put her baby down, but almost impossible as well. He is simply an extension of her body. He suckles whenever he is hungry or thirsty, and sleeps when he is tired. Only in this way can the woman continue her work in much the same way as she did before her child was born.

The baby's new environment is as comforting and familiar as the one that he inhabited prior to his birth. The difference now is the extraordinary range of movement and huge number of sensations that assail him. He is exposed to an enormous number of sights and sounds. He is part of conversations and endless activity. He experiences a full range of movement as his mother bends to plant rice, stretches to pick fruit, rocks to and fro to pound corn, squats to wash clothes in the stream, and fetches water from the well. He feels the warmth of the sun, the breath of the wind and sometimes the rain. He experiences an enormous amount of sensory input, yet always remains in close contact with his mother's body. On some occasions he is cared for by a close relative, perhaps a grandmother or aunt, or even an older brother or sister, but the method of treating him never varies. He is attached to another human's body and he feels the warmth, hears their heartbeat and has all of his senses constantly stimulated.

At night he sleeps nestled against his mother's naked body, probably with another family member, or perhaps several, in the same bed or in very close proximity. He is still able to nurse completely at will, and some studies estimate only 20 minutes of sleep between bursts of sucking. This baby does not awaken fully to nurse, but if he does he is surrounded by the warmth and reassured by the closeness of familiar bodies.

His life continues in much the same fashion until he is mobile, when he is given the opportunity to explore his immediate environment freely. Then he feels the earth between his fingers and toes, and mud on his face. He picks up all the tools and utensils which are part of his carers' lives. When he tires of his exploration he is simply hoisted to his mother's hip or back, where he continues his endless observing and learning. Babies in some societies may be constantly carried for much longer. The feet of Balinese children do not touch the earth at all during their first two years.

At no time is this baby absent from the ebb and flow of life. He has extremely close and constant human company and is very much a part of everything that happens. He never feels neglected, left out, or lonely, and it seems that when he is treated in this manner he has very little cause for complaint. A small baby in traditional cultures rarely cries as a baby in Western society does. He also continues to breast-feed, and will probably do so until well into his fifth year, when weaning is initiated by him. It is then as completely natural and easy as it is inevitable. By then he may have a younger sibling, but he never feels his place usurped by this new baby. He is on the way to being relatively independent by the time the sibling is born. Besides, his mother continues to nurse them both, sleep with them both and, generally, be there for them both. Invariably the loving arms that welcomed him at the time of his birth continue to embrace him very warmly and closely for several years.

Let's look now at the vast difference in our own society's treatment of a new baby.

CHILD CARE IN WESTERN SOCIETY

As we know, in most Western cultures a birth usually takes place in a hospital surrounded by people who are virtual strangers to the mother and her infant. After the warmth and semi-darkness of the womb, the room into which the baby is born is cold and full of bright lights. The newborn's first contact with human flesh is the sensation of being grasped by hands that have no real feeling for him. More detached hands weigh, measure and wash him. They wrap him tightly and hand him back to his mother. He is completely swaddled and has no contact with her warm living flesh. He tries to suckle but if he and his mother have been part of a surgically-assisted delivery, both are stressed by the procedures and may also be suffering from the after effects of drugs. The baby may fall asleep before he has been able to feed properly, and is then taken from his mother while she recovers from the rigours of giving birth.

During the next few days he is returned to her for regular feeds. His mouth is the only part of him that has any contact with her body. He cries a lot, but if his mother has asked for him to be taken to the nursery those cries are lost amongst the cries of all the other newborns, and the attention which he receives there is estimated to be a few minutes in each hour.

If he rooms-in, he is right next to his mother's bed, but in a cold sterile container. She is able to cuddle him more often, but he still feels little of her warmth and hears her heartbeat infrequently. His cries seem to make her nervous. She feeds him, but her tension is transmitted to him. He cries some more and the cycle repeats itself. The new mother is shown how to bathe him, but she lacks confidence, does not hold him securely and he feels as if he is falling. He screams. This makes his mother more nervous still, and once again he senses her tension.

At last this mother and her baby leave the hospital and go home where the woman feels more at ease in her own familiar surroundings. She takes her baby to his nursery that is beautifully decorated with all the things that she and her husband have worked hard for. However, they don't interest the baby one iota. The mother wraps him firmly as she has been shown and puts him in his cot. He feels isolated, lonely, and nothing stimulates his touch receptors, no movement stimulates his position receptors and there is nothing to see in his newborn's field of vision. He falls asleep.

When he wakes he is hungry. He roots around for something to suckle, but there is no comforting nipple near his mouth. He starts to cry, so his mother peers into the cot and picks him up. He enjoys the movement, he can see her face, hear her voice, and she offers him her breast. He begins to suckle and his body relaxes. His mother relaxes too. They sit quietly, he feeds hungrily and feels better now that he is not receiving a constant dose of her stress hormones. Finally, full of milk and at ease in his mother's arms he dozes. But his mother decides that his nappy, which is now wet and dirty, must be changed. The cold air, and the cold hands on his body, wake him and cause him to cry again. His mother wraps him quickly and puts him back in his cot, where he continues to cry for her, before eventually falling asleep—and the cycle repeats itself.

This baby, like all babies, can only cry to signal his needs. His needs are simple. They are for nourishment and comfort from his mother's breast, and for constant and appropriate stimulation, such as that of touch and movement. But this baby is only touched when his nappy is changed and when he is bathed. He only moves when he is picked up for nursing or cuddling. He receives some further sensation of movement when he is taken for a walk in his pram. His mother has learnt to distinguish his hunger cries and feeds him then, but if he cries for any other sort of comfort she puts a dummy in his mouth. Occasionally she simply turns a deaf ear. Someone has told her that babies need to 'exercise their lungs'.

This baby's needs are met intermittently, so he cries a lot. His mother becomes frustrated with his crying. She cannot understand why he is not happy to lie in his cot looking at the pretty coloured frieze and swinging mobile. She becomes particularly irritable, and very tired as well, when she has to get up from her warm bed several times during the night to comfort him. Her husband believes their baby will have to learn that he cannot have his mother whenever he wants her. These parents have read a great deal about child raising and decide to try the 'controlled crying' technique. At first they find it difficult not to respond to their child's cries, but eventually their baby behaves in the manner expected. Because there is no response, he learns that his crying is no use, so he stops.

But these parents have ignored their baby's feelings and their own instincts as well. This leads them to various other parenting choices which are similarly insensitive and detached: playpens, restraints, harnesses, early weaning, then strange baby-sitters and, perhaps, long day care centres, all of which reinforce in subtle ways the things which the baby is beginning to learn. He is learning that he is virtually powerless and unable to influence what happens in his world. He is also learning that his needs and feelings do not seem to matter very much.

His cries have stopped; no one heeds them. His parents are there, but they are remote. However his needs remain; they are unfulfilled. Now his parents can get on with their lives, and they can sleep peacefully through the night, believing that they have trained their baby to be compliant and good. His physical needs are attended to, after a fashion, but in reality their baby has been deprived of almost everything which is truly important for him in his early months of life.

BONDING IS NECESSARY F
ANIMAL SURVIVAL

Bonding is a process that occurs in all mammalian spe
numerous animal researchers have clearly shown that interr
disturbed bonding can have profound effects on the behaviou
a mother and her offspring. For example, if an animal mother i
rated from her babies immediately after birth she may reject t
later, they are reunited. If the separation means that the new r
is unable to lick her young all over, they will not learn to use
bowels or bladder, and if this is the case, they will fail to surviv

Other animal studies show that there is an exquisitely sens
period following the birth when the newborn imprints on whom
(or whatever) is present in the immediate vicinity at the time. In n
instances, the baby will imprint on his mother, but if she is absent th
he will imprint on any object, animate or inanimate, appropriate
inappropriate, which happens to be nearby. This can result in the
formation of quite bizarre bonds between two very disparate animal
species; it can lead to animals strongly bonded to their human carer;
or, sadly, bonded to some inanimate surrogate mother.

The studies also demonstrate what happens when bonding is interrupted or occurs inappropriately, and show that unbonded baby
animals are markedly more fearful, less adventurous and poorly soci-
alised than their bonded counterparts. The animal mother who is not
bonded properly to her babies simply abandons them.

BONDING IS COMPLEX IN
HUMANS

These studies of animals can certainly tell us something about the
importance of the bonding process, although the results may not trans-
late directly to human behaviour. It is not quite so simple to assess the
short and long-term effects of poor or failed bonding in humans, since
the studies designed for animal populations are difficult to conduct and
ethically inappropriate for the human population. As well, humans are
much more complex creatures than any of the animals under study
and the emotional and psychological development of *homo sapiens* is
the result of a large number of interwoven factors which result in

Westside Library
Opening Hours

esday   11.00-8.00
ednesday   11.00-8.00
ursday   11.00-5.00
iday   11.00-5.00
aturday*
.00-1.00   2.00-5.00

* The Library is always
closed the Saturday of
bank holiday weekends

subjective behaviour which may be difficult to interpret or categorise.

Even though direct extrapolation of results is not always possible, the studies have given us some valuable insights into what should, ideally, happen after a woman has given birth. This animal research of Klaus, Kennell, Bowlby and others has been largely responsible for the significant and positive changes that have taken place in birthing practices, and for the improvement in postpartum care of mothers and babies.

BONDING IS BEST
IMMEDIATELY AFTER BIRTH

In our species, it seems that the amazing bonding interplay occurs to best advantage for a period of perhaps no more than twelve hours immediately following the birth. Deferred or less passionate bonding is still possible, but the bonds formed in that critical, immediate postpartum period are very strong. For this reason it's important that all possible attempts are made to ensure that mothers and babies become strongly and appropriately bonded in that period, since this seems to have a positive influence on the mother–baby interaction which extends well beyond the period following the birth. Well-bonded babies appear much more likely to thrive, they seem to have fewer health problems and they also appear to reach their developmental milestones ahead of less well-bonded children.

While human mothers do not need to lick their offspring, they all exhibit an amazing similarity in the manner of fondling and handling their newborn infants. We can safely assume that this touching and caressing is as important in establishing the mother–baby bonds as licking is for other mammals. It appears that the mothers who hold their baby from the moment of birth, who have unlimited skin to skin contact, and who nurse their baby freely and often, have markedly different responses to that baby as he grows. Studies have unequivocally shown that bonded mothers are more likely to continue to breastfeed and also appear to be more patient, more tolerant, and generally in tune with their child's needs. It appears that these women also speak differently to their children and, inevitably, this manner of speaking and relating has a positive influence on the way in which the child responds. The mother's attitude and her child's response establish a cycle of positive reinforcement.

HOW BONDING MAY BE INTERRUPTED

The hours following the birth are critical for establishing strong bonds, and they are hours that cannot be repeated. Given that there is a fairly narrow window of time for bonding to occur to best advantage, it's worth looking at the reasons why it may be interrupted. If drugs have been administered during labour, the perception and instinctive responses of both mother and baby will be quite diminished. A woman who is not active and alert may be unable to hold and nurse her infant, and if her baby is not awake and responsive then bonding is a lot less likely to occur spontaneously. Any surgical intervention during the birth may result in a mother who is in pain, and if she feels that her body has been violated this doesn't augur very well for the early establishment of close bonds. If there were complications during the birth which resulted in a baby suffering from foetal distress, that baby will almost certainly be taken away for resuscitation or observation as soon as he is born. Even though the majority of maternity units now accept the importance of the early postpartum hours for forming deep and lasting bonds, some still play by the old rules and remove the baby for a variety of tests and measurements shortly after the birth.

BONDING TO BEST ADVANTAGE

If you've put into practice all we've talked about in our previous books, then your labour and birth may well be trouble-free and your baby very healthy. Then nothing should take precedence over establishing those bonds. If you have had a natural, unmedicated birth, and if you touch, hold and nurse your infant without interference, the rush of love you feel will be totally overwhelming. This feeling is unique, and is a source of energy and power quite unlike any other emotion ever experienced. Nature has certainly made sure that your baby will be loved and well protected from the moment he enters the world.

After the birth you should hold your naked baby to your body, wait until the umbilical cord has stopped pulsing before it is cut, then caress and nurse your child as you wish. Weighing or measuring doesn't need to be performed during the early postpartum hours. Bathing or washing is also unnecessary, since the coating of vernix rubs into your baby's skin over the next few days and the smell of a newborn baby is incomparably wonderful. Johnson & Johnson tried hard to recreate this smell when they made their baby powder, but unfortunately, in the case of the real thing, the smell lasts no longer than your baby's first bath.

If your birth is medically managed, it's possible that you might experience some initial difficulty in relating to your new baby. Fortunately, humans are very resilient creatures, and if you do not have that all-consuming feeling of love for your baby straight away, it will certainly develop over the next weeks. New mothers—and fathers—may have feelings of detachment, and having to grow to love your baby is simply the result of any interruption to that wonderful interplay of instinctive reactions and responses which occur in the hours immediately after you've given birth. If, for some reason, bonding was interrupted, you need to spend as much time as you can in direct contact with your baby. Nursing him whenever he cries, carrying him close to your body, and taking him into your bed is the best way to do this.

If your maternal feelings don't manifest immediately, there's no need to be alarmed. Not all successful relationships are built on 'love at first sight', and the same is true for mother and child. Give yourself time to get to know your baby, who may seem unfamiliar, have an unexpected appearance or be a different sex from that which you hoped for or anticipated.

If you haven't had children before, you are now experiencing a crash course in becoming a mother. One of the most disturbing feelings for many first-time mothers is that of being in two places at once. Never before have you had the concerns of another human being so much at heart. Your energetic self is now split, and half of it is centred outside yourself, with your child. This can be quite incapacitating, and is perhaps one reason why some new mothers find it difficult to cope. Understanding this process may help you to prevent it being an unsettling experience, and to embrace it as enriching and expansive. One awareness you may have as a result of this is that you are now vulnerable in a new way, through your child, whose wellbeing is as important to you as your own. We can only suggest that you remain confident that life unfolds in rewarding and extraordinary ways, and that the profound joys associated with motherhood will be more than enough to compensate for any grief and suffering.

Some mothers spend the first precious days and weeks of their child's life dwelling on what didn't go right at the birth. This is where those expectations come in again. If you have prepared well, have chosen your caregivers carefully, and are confident that their decisions reflect your own preferences, then any birth that results in a healthy baby is a good birth. It's time now to focus on building your relationship with, and learning how to care for, your new baby. Similarly, try to trust that the rest of your family will manage without your attention for a while, and that your attention is best given to your baby and yourself.

BONDING IS IMPORTANT FOR OTHER FAMILY MEMBERS

While much research has been done on the all important mother–baby bond, the bonds between a father and his baby and between siblings and their new brother or sister are often forgotten. These bonds are just as important and long lasting. We can only wonder at the intensity (or otherwise) of the bonds which formed in those years when the father could only glimpse his child briefly through the nursery window. Similarly, a sibling can't really be expected to form a close attachment to the new baby who comes home from the hospital occupying the arms of the mother which, until that moment, belonged to the older child.

Fortunately, maternity units everywhere now encourage partners not only to be present for the birth of their child, but to act as a support person during labour. However, the presence of siblings at a birth, has yet to achieve the same wide degree of acceptance. (We talked about the presence of partners and children in Chapter 3.)

Of course, as we've just noted, your new baby will make unprecedented demands on your time and energy and this may result in your family feeling uncared for and unsupported. Your partner may genuinely fear that he has been supplanted in your affections, and even feel jealous of the baby. He may resent the new demands being made on him to support you both financially and with time and energy. You need to be aware of this, and make sure that you share your child with him. It's his baby too—and he needs to feel that he is included in this incredibly strong bond that is developing. This is especially important as your other joint activities, especially those that are recreational, will be interrupted and pushed aside for more urgent concerns. This is true for your other children as well, who also need to be included in caring for your baby, and given their own time with you in order to feel that they are still important. You'll need to trust other members of your family to carry and hold your baby close.

Another change in your relationship may be your attitude to sex. This concerns many new mothers (and fathers!) but it's very natural, and is all part of Mother Nature's way of spacing children.

At first, you will probably feel genitally 'exhausted' and need time to recover physically. Then you may well find that your physical and sensual response is centred on the breast, and your developing relationship with your nursing child. The high levels of prolactin present at this time will tend to delay ovulation, and this is all part of nature's plan to make sure you have time to recover nutritionally, and bond with your first child, before conceiving the next. An ideal gap between children is at least two years, if the subsequent children are to have their nutritional and emotional needs met.

During this time of no ovulation, because your hormones never reach the libidinous peaks of mid-cycle, when you would normally be fertile and seeking a mate, your sex drive may also be reduced. This is still part of the divine plan, as the more frequently you are sexually active, the faster your fertility returns. So don't worry, you're not the first couple to experience these changes, and things will return to normal in their own good time.

Another concern for some women, if they have stopped work to have their baby, is their lack of financial independence. This can be as much a worry for you as the responsibility of providing support is for your partner, and may be exacerbated by anxiety about job security. Again, forewarned is forearmed, and the more you can discuss and arrange in advance, the less you will be affected. Your relationships at work may change, even if you return to your job soon after the birth, because your baby will become your major concern.

Working mothers have huge demands on them, but hopefully you will have organised the support you need to make it all possible. Just don't underestimate the strong emotional needs both you and your baby have to be together. Extended families are certainly the best support possible, and you may find that your relationship with your own mother enters a new fruitful stage as you share with her the joys of children. In fact you'll be amazed at the strong connection you now feel with all mothers everywhere. Women with whom you may have previously felt no bond may suddenly become important to you in your shared experiences. You'll share smiles of conspiracy with other women in the street, as they struggle with strollers and shopping bags, soothe their crying baby, or just walk along smiling blissfully with their baby in their arms.

WHY IS TOUCH SO IMPORTANT?

Your skin is your largest sensory organ as well as the most primitive. The sense most closely associated with the skin, the sense of touch, is the earliest to develop in the human embryo. This means touch is an extremely important sense, for the earlier a function develops, the more fundamental it appears to be. A human being can spend his life deaf and blind, and lacking the senses of taste or smell, but he cannot survive at all without the functions performed by the skin.

The foetus receives stimulation of all the cutaneous (skin) receptors during its time in utero, and during labour this stimulation increases dramatically as the uterine contractions increase in intensity. At the time of birth these receptors are further stimulated, as your baby makes his journey down the birth canal. This stimulation is vitally important, for it appears to prime your baby's respiratory, circulatory, eliminative, digestive and endocrine systems for their existence outside the womb. It is also essential for the proper functioning of the nervous system, and lack of this stimulation seems to affect how well many senses develop. Research has shown that if a baby receives none of the squeezing, pummelling and general pressure on his skin which is the legacy of a vaginal birth, he appears to lag behind in many stages of his development. If your medical history means that you can't avoid a Caesarean, you should at least discuss with your doctor the possibility of letting labour begin spontaneously, and proceed for as long as possible. This means that your baby will receive at least some degree of sensory stimulation.

Touch is something that every human being needs, and must have in abundance if he is to develop into an emotionally stable and healthy individual. Studies made long ago of orphan children who were never touched showed that these children did not thrive. Many of the foundlings in orphanages who received no human handling at all succumbed to a condition called 'marasmus', which means wasting away for no reason. To state things simply, these infants died for want of human touch. A much more recent study carried out in the USA has linked an epidemic of adolescent suicides (1975–1978) with the growth to adolescence of the first very premature babies to be treated in neonatal intensive care units. It was found that these adolescents had suffered 400 per cent more perinatal complications as infants than the average child. Babies treated in the early days of these units were almost totally sensorially deprived: they were isolated in an incubator or humidicrib and received almost no human touch at all. Today, staff who work in these units have a far greater understanding of the sensorial needs of 'premie' babies.

These findings also tell us something about the needs of your normal, healthy, full term baby. Touching is enormously comforting, and your baby has an exquisitely sensitive need to be touched. By simply carrying him close, you can ensure that all the touch receptors on his body are constantly stimulated. Almost unconsciously you will touch his face, hold his hands, stroke his head, and caress his body. It's very easy for you to satisfy this fundamental biological need if you carry your child attached to your body in some fashion.

As well as carrying him close, you can learn some simple techniques of baby massage, which is something that mothers in traditional societies have regularly practised. As you massage him, you'll be able to see and feel him physically relax. What you cannot feel or see is your baby's brain becoming denser, but his cerebral cortex actually becomes heavier with this sort of stimulation. As well, when you touch your child constantly in this fashion, he will be aware of the feeling of warmth and caring which your hands impart, and he will be much more likely to return the warmth and caring when he is able.

THE PHYSICAL BENEFITS OF BONDING

Your new baby must have all his senses stimulated if he is to grow and to learn. In particular, he must experience almost constant movement if his nervous system is to develop and function properly. Nature has devised a truly perfect system, for if you carry your infant in your arms or close to your body he will automatically be exposed to a full range of movement and to all sorts of other sensations as well.

As you go about your daily activities, your baby is in the perfect position to observe everything that you do. He is very sensitive to smells, he will be aware of all your conversations, and he receives constant tactile stimulation as your body moves against his. His specialised (proprio-) receptors receive signals that tell him about the position of his body, which way it is aligned, and its size and shape. As you move, the vestibular mechanism in his inner ear is stimulated. This stimulation is vital for his balance and in fact for the integration of all those messages he receives from his eyes, nose, ears, skin and other sensory receptors. If your baby is carried as an extension of your body you will probably find that he catnaps or sleeps in brief stretches of about 20 minutes. When he is awake, he may nurse or may simply be happy to drink in all the sensations surrounding him.

By contrast, the baby who lies in a cot or a pram seems to sleep for much longer periods between wakeful ones. Yet we generally think of this docile, endlessly sleeping infant as the 'good baby' and are dismayed by or worry about the child who seems to sleep for much shorter periods. But you should remember that the child who is awake for much of the day is constantly learning. By contrast, if you put your baby down in some sort of bed, cot or baby carriage you are denying him countless learning experiences and, usually, since he lacks adequate or appropriate stimulation, he simply goes to sleep or cries for attention.

Your breastfed baby also continues to receive sensorial stimulation denied to his bottle-fed counterpart. As your baby nurses and shifts from the left to the right breast and vice versa he is receiving information which will later be important in the establishment of his 'handedness'. As he grows older he will inevitably learn to fondle your free nipple while he nurses from the other. It seems that this action, which resembles some sort of constant five finger exercise, will have positive implications for his later fine motor development and coordination. And finally, the skin-to-skin contact he receives while you nurse him stimulates his tactile senses. But that's just one of the myriad benefits of feeding your baby the way that nature intended! More of the others in our next book.

MAKING THE BEST OF A DIFFICULT BEGINNING

Despite believing passionately in the value of, and need for, a strong bonding experience with your baby, you might, like Francesca with her first child and Jan with her second, find yourself in the difficult position of being unable to fulfil your goals as fully as you'd like. Your baby may be in an intensive care unit, or he (or perhaps you) may be unable to leave the hospital because of medical requirements. If this is the case, you will need to focus as positively as you can on grasping every opportunity for bonding, and offering your baby the emotional security he craves and needs. This is important for your own emotional stability and wellbeing too.

First, you can insist that you stay in the hospital, so you can be as close and available to your baby as possible. This is especially important if you live a considerable distance away. If this isn't a viable option (hospitals are pretty crowded places these days), try to find some alternative accommodation in the immediate vicinity.

The second—and vitally important—contribution you can make to your child's health, wellbeing and progress out of the hospital is to make sure your baby gets your breast milk exclusively, particularly the colostrum that is produced in the first few days after birth. Right from the word go make it clear that you do not want your child given any supplementary feeding. If your baby is too small, weak or sick to suckle, you can express your milk and have it fed to him through whatever delivery mechanism is available (normally a tube directly to his stomach).

This is especially important if he has been born prematurely. The composition of your breast milk is different in this situation and nature has made sure that it is ideally suited to the needs of a 'premie' baby. Expressing will also ensure that your milk supply is well established and able to support your baby adequately when you take him home. (If you're expressing more than your baby can take, you may be able to donate it to the hospital milk bank.) A study carried out on 424 pre-term infants in the UK clearly showed that the diet fed to a premature baby for an average of four weeks after birth had a significant effect on his IQ in later life and also affected the incidence of cerebral palsy. We're sure that these ill effects are only the tip of the iceberg and that many other problems could (and will) be shown to be attributed to inappropriate nutrition for 'premies', so you need to be very sure that the medical and nursing staff are quite clear about your wishes and that they comply with them.

You must also hold or touch your child as often as possible. Your hormones and your emotions are in such a state of flux at this time and all your senses and responses are so well primed for holding your baby in your arms that to be unable to do so can produce an almost unbearable physical ache. But, not surprisingly, you'll actually feel much better if you're close to your baby and can touch him in whatever way possible. These days the nursing staff in neonatal units are very aware of the importance of mother–baby contact and will make whatever efforts they can to facilitate this. Some hospitals encourage skin-to-skin contact for as much time as possible, even if your baby has monitors attached to him. Don't be afraid to ask to nurse your baby. Let him snuggle against your chest, even if he is hooked up to tubes and breathing apparatus. You might also be able to carry him around in a sling for short spells. Studies show that sick or premature babies who receive this type of 'kangaroo care' actually have improved growth and faster recovery rates than those babies who receive little touching and holding.

Jan hardly left the neonatal unit during Michael's 48-hour visit and was able to touch him and hold him for a good proportion of that time. Francesca stayed in the hospital for three weeks, until her son was able to come home. Despite the fact that he was so tiny that he could nestle in one of her cupped hands, she spent nearly the whole time in the intensive care ward touching, holding and talking to her baby.

Don't be afraid to ask for whatever physical contact is possible. If this is impossible, or if contact must be restricted for some reason, your hospital may use a 'doughnut'. These are soft circular cushions resembling a draught stopper which, when wrapped around your baby, can give him the feeling of having a boundary (such as your uterus, or your arms) around him, that he can kick against. This device can help him to feel more secure and settled and to feed and sleep better.

If your baby is confined to a humidicrib, you can still stroke and caress him through the sterile gloves that are inset in the side of the crib. Although it may be heart-breaking if you are unable to touch him directly, you can still send him reassuring and stimulating messages that he is not alone in the world. You can talk, hum, sing and chant to him too. He has been accustomed to hearing your voice all through the pregnancy. He's completely unaccustomed to the relative silence of the humidicrib, where only mechanical and impersonal sounds reach him. He will respond to the emotional overtones in your voice, to the rhythms of speech, to the encouragement and love that you express even if you are unable to demonstrate these physically by holding him.

Your own emotional state may be very fragile at this time—you may be frightened for your baby, and if he is your first, scared by the strength of your response, and how vulnerable you are, through him, to processes somewhat outside of your control. Make sure that you are emotionally supported, so that you are able to express those positive feelings of love, comfort and encouragement. When you're not able to be present with your baby, see if your partner, your parents, your siblings or your friends can stand in for you. Make sure that your baby is left alone as little as possible. Also keep a constant flow of questions and answers going with the medical staff. This way you'll be confident that your baby is not only receiving the best care, but also minimal medication and medical intervention, and reassured that you'll be able to take him home as soon as possible.

Usually, your child will gain strength and health quite fast, and your contact with him can increase all the time. Just make sure you are always taking advantage of the opportunities available to you. When you finally get him home, you can make up for lost time. It's important that you then have the necessary support so that you can give him your full attention, just as you would if you had only just given birth.

Francesca's sons, both the first who was in the 'premie' ward for three weeks and the second who was with her from birth onwards, developed a great taste for the family bed, which had to grow considerably as they did. 'Musical beds' was a favourite night-time activity as they got older, with each dawn finding a different combination of tumbled bodies in different locations. Extended breastfeeding of both her sons also contributed to their emotional security and development, and though those first three weeks still cause her heartache when she thinks back, she's confident that her compensatory efforts have filled the gap, and that her first son recovered from the experience completely. The memories of the early days following the birth of Janette's second son bring her heartache too, but all she did before and after the birth have left Michael apparently unfazed by the experience. In fact, it seems that those days were more of a challenge to all the beliefs that Jan held dear than a challenge to her son.

So don't be too downhearted if your bonding experience isn't ideal. The overwhelming love that you feel for your baby *can* find expression and he *can* receive it, whatever the circumstances, and if you can find ways to express it to him, then the rest will follow.

Your baby's wellbeing will be your major concern for many years. The most important gift you can give him is your constant presence and your unconditional love, but feeding him well and making sure his environment is free of toxicity are important factors too. If you've been following our recommendations all along, your baby's off to a head start in all departments but now you're ready for the next stage—breastfeeding. Since our coverage here has been necessarily brief, this is where we leave you while we rush off and finish our next book that tells you all about this topic (and what comes afterwards too). In the meantime, if you stick to the same healthy diet and lifestyle that we recommend for before conception and during pregnancy, and if you keep taking those supplements as we suggest, your breastfeeding experience should be trouble free and long-term. But you'll still want to know what to do about timing feeds (don't), weaning (don't), and issues like introducing solids (just leave it as late as possible) and LOTS MORE . . .

SO JUST STAY TUNED—AND WE'LL BE BACK BEFORE YOU KNOW IT!

How to use natural remedies and treatments

Where we've recommended natural remedies and treatments throughout the book we've drawn on many traditions—some, such as herbal medicine, have been used by midwives and 'wise women' for centuries. Acupuncture and pressure points also have ancient and traditional use. Homoeopathy, hypnotherapy, aromatherapy, flower essences and reflexology, which are more recently developed modalities, though based on folklore, have all been shown through clinical trials to be of assistance in achieving an easier birth and a more rapid recovery. Body-centred therapies such as osteopathy and massage are also effective in relieving a number of conditions.

All these natural treatments and remedies have the advantage of being kinder to your body and mind than medical drugs and, though it would be foolish to believe that they can do no harm, if they are used within informed guidelines, or by professionals, they are very safe. Frequently they can address problems for which orthodox medicine has no answer, or provide support for recovery if drugs or surgery are required.

Although some of the advice we give in this book can be used for self-help, whenever possible you should find an appropriate health professional to guide and support you. Diagnosis, choice of appropriate remedy and dosage are some of the decisions that are best left to a qualified practitioner who will also be able to distinguish between a situation that may be amenable to a natural approach, and one needing medical management. Refer to Contacts and Resources if you have no personal recommendations or referrals.

Although there are some herbs, pressure points, essential oils and other natural treatments that are contraindicated during pregnancy, many of these can be used in the last few weeks approaching the birth. We have indicated where a remedy or treatment is not appropriate for use in early or late pregnancy. Otherwise you can be assured that there is no evidence of any possible problem associated with its use, though occasionally there may be a very slight risk which is justified in terms of the benefits to be gained. If, despite our recommendations, you are in any doubt about a course of action, please consult your midwife or health practitioner and be guided by them.

HOW TO USE NATURAL REMEDIES AND TREATMENTS

Nutrition

If you eat well and take your supplements every day this will help you to avoid many, if not all, of the problems we discuss. However, should the need arise, some nutrients can be used therapeutically in dosages greater than usual daily requirements. Where we have listed single nutrients, or even a range of them, as specific treatment for a condition, this doesn't change the continuing need for a balanced diet and comprehensive supplementation. It may, however, be necessary to increase the dosage of a certain nutrient temporarily. Alternatively you may find that you are already taking the required amount as part of your daily regimen. A qualified naturopath, or practitioner trained in the use of nutritional therapies can recommend the most appropriate form of any nutrient.

Herbal medicine

Information on herbal medicine is very comprehensive these days. Not only is there a substantial and growing body of scientific research into the constituents and effects of herbs, but also the advantage of experience gathered over many centuries of traditional use.

Herbal remedies can be used in one of two ways. Preferably, you should consult a qualified medical herbalist (who may, in some cases, also be a medical doctor). A herbalist will probably prescribe liquid preparations (fluid extracts or tinctures) which are the most concentrated and flexible form, especially when making up individual formulae. They may also prescribe tablets or capsules, and, for some conditions, give you the dried herb to make into an infusion or tea. With any prescription you are given, the practitioner will also set the appropriate dose (or dose range).

If you are following our advice for self-help, it's easier, and safer, to use herbal infusions, which can be made according to the following instructions:

How to make a herbal tea or infusion

1. For every 30 g (two tablespoons) of herb, pour on 600 mL of boiling water.
2. Let it steep (infuse) for at least 15 minutes to get the full benefit of the active ingredients.
3. Strain.
4. Drink a cupful three times daily (during late pregnancy).
5. Make a fresh brew every day, use it within 24 hours, or refrigerate.

While infusions are not, in most cases, as potent as the preparations you will receive from a herbalist, they can still be very effective, and in some cases are the preferred form. Although you will find you can treat yourself easily if the condition is mild, any severe or continuing problem requires professional diagnosis and treatment.

You will also find many herbal medicines in tablet or capsule form in health food shops, and these should have clear directions (and cautions for pregnancy) on the label. While staff in these shops may be able to advise you, we strongly recommend that you check all herbal preparations, whatever form they may take, with a qualified herbalist, or against our recommendations, regarding their safety (bearing in mind the stage of your pregnancy).

Pressure points

Pressure points can be used in a variety of ways. In reflexology treatments the finger or thumb is used to put pressure on points on the foot. The following diagrams show all the points and areas that are recommended for various conditions throughout the book.

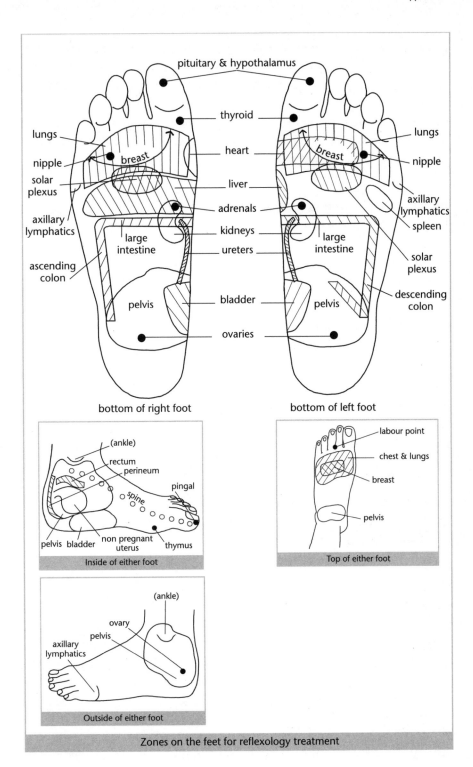

pituitary & hypothalamus

thyroid

lungs

nipple

solar plexus

axillary lymphatics

ascending colon

heart

breast

liver

adrenals

kidneys

ureters

large intestine

large intestine

pelvis

bladder

pelvis

ovaries

lungs

nipple

axillary lymphatics

spleen

solar plexus

descending colon

bottom of right foot

bottom of left foot

(ankle)

rectum

perineum

pingal

spine

pelvis bladder

non pregnant uterus

thymus

Inside of either foot

labour point

chest & lungs

breast

pelvis

Top of either foot

(ankle)

ovary

pelvis

axillary lymphatics

Outside of either foot

Zones on the feet for reflexology treatment

Acupressure may involve the use of needles, heat (Moxibustion—see Chapter 7) or even laser or electrical stimulation to trigger the release of 'chi', or energy, at a point. Acupressure, or Shiatsu, is the practice of stimulating these points through manual pressure. Acupressure points are formed on various meridians, or energy pathways, around the body, and we've included a diagram when we've recommended the use of a particular point.

How to stimulate an acupressure point

First, find the point as accurately as you can, then apply pressure in the appropriate way. Choose from the three methods below, unless specific instructions are given:

Calming

Cover the point with the palm of the hand, or gently stroke, for about two minutes. This method should be used when over-activity is involved, for example in the treatment of stress.

Tonifying

Apply stationary (or clockwise) pressure for two minutes. This pressure can be slowly increased as your tolerance of any discomfort increases (points relating to an organ or condition in need of treatment may often be tender). If you press too hard straight away, you may tense. Pressure that increases gradually can be better tolerated, and more easily built up to effective levels. This method should be used for sluggish or depressed conditions.

Dispersing

Apply moving pressure, such as a circular anticlockwise motion, or a pumping action in and out, on the point. The pressure can be begun fairly deep, then brought up to the surface. Take care to keep the area relaxed, and increase the pressure on successive treatments as your tolerance improves. This method should be used when there is congestion.

As with herbal medicine, you'll get the best results if you use the services of a qualified practitioner, who may also be able to help you with other problems that we have not listed.

Homoeopathy

Homoeopathy works by introducing minute amounts of herbal or mineral substances to the body, which trigger a response of self-healing, either in the body or in the mind. As the amounts used are infinitesimally small (and may not even be traceable on analysis) they have no potential for toxicity and are therefore an excellent choice for the pregnant or birthing mother, especially as their effect can be powerful and immediate.

Although we've recommended a wide range of remedies for you to choose from, expert help is always preferable since self-diagnosis can be tricky, especially when you are under stress (as you are during labour). Homoeopathy works best if you use a single remedy. This needs to be chosen carefully and if you have no access to a homoeopath, it's best to get one of your support people to familiarise themselves with the different options.

Aromatherapy

Essential oils can be very effective in pregnancy and during labour. However some should be avoided, so use only those that we suggest, or get advice (or treatment) from a trained aromatherapist. In the hands of a skilled practitioner, they are even more effective if used on specific points during a massage. You can also incorporate them in a self-help massage routine. Although in some cultures it's common to ingest essential oils as therapy, this is definitely not an option we recommend in pregnancy, or without professional supervision. The best ways for you to use the oils are as follows:

How to use essential oils

Vaporisation or inhalation

Vaporisers or oil burners use either a candle or electric current as a source of heat. Generally, about six drops of the oil are added to a small amount of water in the bowl of the burner, though sometimes, with electric vaporisers, the oil is added directly to the heated surface. Alternatively, you can simply add the oil to a bowl containing about a litre of hot water, and keep it warm over a radiator. Leaning over the bowl, with a towel forming a tent over your head, allows more direct inhalation. This is a useful technique if you want the decongestant effect of steam on your respiratory system. You might prefer to place a few drops of oil on a hanky or your pillowslip, and there are also some devices that fit over a light bulb.

Topical application

Oils can be applied during a massage, or directly onto your skin at a specific point. For a massage, add a few drops to a vegetable oil base (try sweet almond, grapeseed or any good quality massage oil) in the ratio of one drop of essential oil to each 2 mL of base oil. You can also use a base cream (try vitamin E cream), with one drop of oil required for each 4 g of cream. If you know of a particular point that will benefit from a direct application, you can use one drop of the undiluted oil.

Compresses

Hot or cold compresses, with the added benefit of essential oils, can be helpful during labour. Disperse a few drops of oil over the surface of a bowl containing very hot or ice cold water. Use a soft cloth to collect the oil from the surface, lightly squeeze out excess moisture and place the cloth over the affected area (probably your abdomen or lower back).

In your bath

If you find baths relaxing during the latter stages of pregnancy, or if you plan to make use of a bath or birth pool during labour, this method may be helpful. You will need a dispersing base so that the oil doesn't collect in droplets on the top of the bath water. You can buy fragrance free, dispersing bath oil and add your own preferred aromas. You'll only need about six drops of essential oil in an egg-cupful of dispersing oil. If this is not available, you can use vodka or full-cream milk as a base.

Flower essences

Bach or Bush flower essences can be prescribed and dispensed by your health practitioner, or you can find them in your health food shop. They are non-toxic and very safe, though an accurate diagnosis makes for more effective treatment. Since everyone usually feels they need most, if not all, of the remedies, self-diagnosis can be difficult. If you don't have access to a practitioner who knows the remedies well, ask a close friend or your partner to help you choose. (See also Chapter 7).

Other therapies

A professional massage can be a blissful experience, as well as therapeutic, but using massage as a self-help measure can also be useful. Yoga is best practised with a qualified teacher. Hypnotherapy and osteopathy should only be performed by a trained practitioner (although a hypnotherapist can teach you how to use self-hypnosis).

In tune with

the moon

We mentioned in the text that the length of your pregnancy is, like that of your menstrual cycle, determined by the lunar month. Women who practise Natural Fertility Management are aware of this connection, as they are aware of how their own personal lunar bio-rhythm can affect their fertility and the timing of their ovulation. Natural methods for timing conception, or avoiding it, are more effective if this personal lunar cycle is taken into account, with the woman experiencing raised fertility if she ovulates at the same point in the lunar month at which she was born. If this does not occur, there seems to be an increased tendency at this personal lunar 'birthday' for a spontaneous ovulation to occur, and many an unexplained conception, and confusion over dates, can be resolved when this cycle is taken into account. This cycle also seems to influence the timing of birth, and the following story beautifully illustrates this ancient connection between the moon, women and fertility.

This delightful study is from a student of Natural Fertility Management, a woman who had previously used mucus and temperature charting, but was learning about the lunar cycle for the first time. She had kept extensive and accurate records of all her many children's conceptions and births, and we calculated a 'retrospective' lunar chart for her, giving her personal 'lunar peak' times, relating to her own bio-rhythm, over these years. There was a tendency to twins in her family, so it may be that she was particularly susceptible to the influence of the lunar cycle, as this 'additional' potentially fertile time has been found to be responsible for the conception of non-identical twins.

The following is her fascinating story, which may be interesting to those of you who have previously had arguments with your doctor about conception and 'due' dates.

During a recent Natural Fertility Management course, I was interested to learn of the effect of the lunar cycle on fertility. This was perhaps an explanation for the otherwise unexpected arrival of my two youngest children, who were conceived while we were using the Billings Method. Our daughter, now nine, was conceived 9–10 days after I believed I had ovulated ('spinn', or fertile, mucus followed by a clear sustained temperature rise lasting over one week). Our son, now nearly four, was conceived *18 days* after I had recorded ovulation symptoms and a rise in basal temperature. In addition to avoiding all sexual contact near ovulation, we were using a barrier method at all other times. Throughout the pregnancies, I had experienced long running problems convincing health professionals that my babies were due later than the dates assumed from the date of my last period (and that I was not stupid, vague, lying or having an extramarital relationship!). Interestingly, both babies arrived well past their official 'due dates': our daughter, 4300 g, '10 days late' but with no signs of postmaturity; and our son was induced, '18 days overdue' weighing 4600 g but with no signs of postmaturity.

Francesca kindly provided me with some retrospective lunar cycle charts so that I could see if there was a link. I was also interested in seeing if the lunar angle return was connected to the onset of labour. The results? Quite amazing! I was able to remember these children's conception dates (a bit hard to forget when there had been so much debate about it during the pregnancies) and both correlated beautifully with the lunar cycle. It solved a mystery for us. Awareness of the lunar cycle may have prevented these pregnancies—though I would hasten to add that we all love these two 'lunar children' dearly and would not change anything about them or their births at all. We believe that they are special people who were really meant to be here. It may be interesting to add that both these children were conceived while we were both 'shellshocked' by the deaths of close family members. While I do not have any firm opinions on reincarnation, our daughter has many strong similarities in personality, talents and interests to her grandmother who died so close to her conception.

At the time, I wondered if a second ovulation was possible in some cycles. This idea was dismissed as ludicrous by an obstetrician, but I do wonder, especially in light of my strong family history of non-identical twins who have been born with significant gaps in birth weight and maturity.

The conception dates of our two older sons also tallied well with the lunar cycle—I was able to remember these easily as they coincided with easily remembered dates such as our wedding anniversary and Easter. In both cases, this was probably lunar cycle and mid-cycle ovulation being synchronised.

Of these four children mentioned, spontaneous onset of labour coincided with the lunar cycle in two cases. In the other two, it didn't. I did, however, experience 'false labour' significantly enough to spend the night at the birth centre. I could remember the date too—it was my niece's birthday and she was disappointed that her cousin missed her birthday by a week. It would be interesting to see if other parents or midwives have noticed the effect of the lunar cycle on uterine irritability.

Contacts and resources

Francesca and Jan offer the following services that can augment and update the information in this book.

Books

- *Healthy Parents, Better Babies* by Francesca Naish and Janette Roberts, Gill & Macmillan
- *Healthy Lifestyle, Better Pregnancy* by Francesca Naish and Janette Roberts, Gill & Macmillan

These books are available through all good book stores or through the internet.

- *Natural Fertility: The Complete Guide to Avoiding or Achieving Conception* by Francesca Naish, Sally Milner Publishing, $AU33.00 (plus postage).
- *The Lunar Cycle* by Francesca Naish, Nature & Health Books, $AUS13.20 (plus postage).

For the above books, send credit card details (Visa/Mastercard/Bankcard) to:
Natural Fertility Management
PO Box 786
Castlemaine VIC 3450
Australia
Ph: (61–3) 5472 4922, Fax: (61–3) 5470 5766
Or order through: www.fertility.com.au

Foresight Association

Jan is the Australian representative of Foresight, The UK Association for the Promotion of Preconceptual Care. Members receive regular newsletters with updated research results. Fully referenced booklets are available, detailing the adverse effects on reproduction of the following: alcohol, tobacco, zinc deficiency, manganese deficiency, food additives, genito-urinary infections, lead and agrochemicals. The Foresight video 'Preparing for the Healthier Baby' (running time 85 minutes) is suitable for viewing by preconception couples. Information about Foresight practitioners and hair analysis (for toxic metals) is also available. Contact:

Foresight (Registered Charity No: 279160)
Mrs. Peter Barnes
28 The Paddock, Godalming, Surrey GU7 1XD
Ph: (01483) 427839
Hours 9.30am-6.00pm
Website: www.foresight-preconception.org.uk

Lane Cove Wellness Centre

Jan is an associate at one of the first centres of its type in Australia. The centre offers wellness programs for preconception, pregnancy, breast-feeding and vitality and longevity. For information about:

- Nutritional supplements that fulfill the recommendations in Jan and Francesca's books

- Postal/online programs

- TUBETRAIN exercise system—complete with workout video, contact:

Lane Cove Wellness Centre
152 Burns Bay Road
Lane Cove NSW 2066
Australia
Ph: (61–2) 9420 4959, Fax: (61–2) 9418 6846
Website: www.wellnesscentre.com.au
email: janroberts@wellnesscentre.com.au

Payment for nutritional supplements, TUBETRAIN system and postal programs can be made by Visa, Mastercard or Bankcard.

Natural Fertility Management

Francesca is the director of Natural Fertility Management which is currently commencing operations in the United Kingdom, and offers the following services through the NFM website:

www.fertility.com.au

Or you can write to:

The International Coordinator
Natural Fertility Management
PO Box 786
CASTLEMAINE VIC 3450
AUSTRALIA

for an NFM contact near you, or details of our postal services.

Natural Fertility Management offers programs for:

- Contraception
- Conscious conception
- Overcoming fertility problems

These programs can be easily followed through our correspondence service, which gives detailed instruction in the use of mucus, temperature and lunar methods, as well as extensive naturopathic and herbal advice for reproductive health. If you wish for more individual recommendations, there is an option to order personal advice, as well as the kit. The kit includes:

- A copy of the book *Natural Fertility: A complete guide to avoiding or achieving conception* (or rebate on proof of purchase).

- An audio cassette with:
  1. Instructions for contraception or conception and use of lunar cycle charts, and
  2. Relaxation techniques, visualisations, and suggestions to assist the synchronization of cycles, increase confidence and motivation, promote reproductive health and general well-being, and deal with stress. In the conception kit there are also suggestions for a healthy conception, pregnancy and birth.

- Blank sympto-thermal charts for recording mucus and temperature and other observations for each menstrual cycle.

- Individual computer-calculated lunar charts showing the potentially fertile times on your personal bio-rhythmic fertility cycle for the next ten years.

- Current year Moon Calendar, showing moon phase present on each day of the year.

- Time zone calculator, to adjust times given on your personal lunar chart for different time zones.

- Attractively bound printed notes for conception or contraception, taking you through the first few months, cycle by cycle.

Options
- For postal or internet clients: detailed written personal advice, including appropriate naturopathic remedies.

- For conscious conception clients: sex selection calculations and advice.

- For clients overcoming fertility problems: male lunar chart, male relaxation and suggestion tape.

Please send for order forms, current fees or addresses of Natural Fertility Management accredited counsellors to the International Coordinator, at the address above, or through the website.

Natural Fertility Management Counsellor Training
Seminars will be conducted by Francesca Naish to train health professionals in Natural Fertility Management techniques and the 'Better Babies' program of preconception health care. All accredited counsellors have access to Natural Fertility Management kits for their clients. For details and dates of training in the United Kingdom, contact the International Coordinator, as above.

Other Contacts and Resources

The following list has been compiled to support the information in Jan and Francesca's books. Further details of other associations, health centres and support groups can be found at:

http://www.foresight-preconception.org.uk

http://www.babyonline.com

Action Against Allergy, 24-26 High Street, Hampton Hill, Middlesex TW12 1PD

Action on Smoking and Health (ASHO), 10 Gloucester Place, London W1, Ph: 020 7935 3519

Active Birth Centre, 25 Bickerton Road, London N19 5JT, Ph: 0171 561 9006, Fax: 0171 561 9007

Active Birth Movement, 52 Dartmouth Park Road, London NW5 1SL

Aqua (Laundry) Washing Balls, FREEPHONE 0800 026 0220

Aqualink, 5 Albion Parade, Albion Road, Stoke Newington, London N16 9LD, Ph: 020 7275 9099 (water filters and water deliveries)

Association for Breastfeeding Mothers, Sydenham Green Health Centre, 26 Holmshaw Close, Sydenham, London SE26 4TH

The Association for Holistic Biodynamic Massage Therapy, 20 Oak Drive, Larksfield, Aylesford, Kent ME20 6NU, Ph: 0173 287 5605

The Association for the Improvement of Maternity Services (AIMS) 40 Kingswood Avenue, London NW6 6LS, Ph: 0181 960 5585

Association of Natural Medicine, 19a Collingwood Road, Witham, Essex CM8 2DY, Ph: 0137 650 2762

Association of Radical Midwives (ARM) 62 Greetby Hill, Ormskirk, Lancashire L39 2DT, Ph / Fax: 01695 572776, email: arm@radmid. demon.co.uk

Association of Reflexologists, 27 Old Gloucester Street, London WC1N 3XX, Ph: 0870 567 3320

Biocare, Lakeside, 180 Lifford Lane, Kings Norton, Birmingham B30 3NT, Ph: 0121 433 3727, email: 100574,1017@compuserve.com (nutritional supplements)

Biodynamic Agriculture Association (BDAA) The Painswick Inn Project, Gloucester Street, Stroud, Gloucestershire GL5 IQ6, Ph: 0145 375 9501

British Homoeopathic Association, 27a Devonshire Street, London W1N 1RJ

British Institute for Allergy and Environmental Therapy, Llangwyryfon, Aberystwyth, Dyfed SY23 4EY, Ph: 0197 424 1376

British Osteopathic Association, 8–10 Bolston Place, Marylebone, London NW1 6QH, Ph: 020 7262 5250/1128

British Psychological Society, St Andrews House, 48 Princess Road East, Leicester LE1 7DR, Ph: 0116 254 9568, email: enquiry@ops.org.uk

British Society for Allergy and Environmental Medicine Foundation, PO Box 28, Totton, Southampton

British Society for Nutritional Medicine, PO Box 3AP, London W1A 3AP

Cantassium Company, Green Farm, Larkhall Grove Labs, 225 Putney Bridge Rd, London SW15 2PY (nutritional supplements)

Centre for Alternative Technology (CAT), Machynlleth, Powys SY20 9AZ, Ph: 0165 470 2400, email: media@catinfo.demon.co.uk

Central Register of Advanced Hypnotherapists, Box 14526, London N2 2WG, Ph: 020 7354 9938

CHILD, Charter House, 43 St Leonards Road, Bexhill-on-Sea, East Sussex TN40 1JA, Ph: 0142 473 2361 (infertility support group)

Diagnostic (UK), Cultech Ltd, York Chambers, York Street, Swansea SA1 3NJ, FREEPHONE 0800 731 5655, email: cultech@btinternet.com (diagnostic and allergy tests and practitioner referral)

Ecos Organic Paints, Lakeland Paints, Ph: 0153 973 2866

Exploring Parenthood, 4 Ivory Place, Treadgold Street, London W11 4BP, Ph: 0171 221 9951, Fax: 0171 221 5501

Family Planning Association, 27–35 Mortimer Street, London W1N 7RJ Ph: 171 636 7866

Fertility Education Trust, National Secretariat, 24 Selly Wick Drive, Selly Park, Birmingham B29 7JH

Fertility UK, Clitherow House, 1 Blythe Mews, Blythe Road, London W14 ONW, Ph: 020 7371 1341, email: jknight@fertilityuk.org (natural family planning)

FPA UK, 27–35 Mortimer Street, London W1N 7RJ, Ph: 020 7636 7866 (natural family planning)

Fresh Water Filter Company, Gem House, 895 High Road, Chadwell Heath, Essex RM6 4HL, email: mail@freshwaterfilter.demon.co.uk

Guild of Complementary Practitioners, Liddell House, 6 Liddell Close, Finchampstead, Berkshire RG40 4NS, Ph: 0118 973 5757, email: info@gcpnet.com

International Academy of Oral Medicine and Toxicology, Tony Newby President, 72 Harley Street, London W1N 1AE, Ph: 020 7580 3168 (holistic dentists)

International Federation of Aromatherapists (IFA), Stamford House, 2/4 Chiswick High Road, London W4 1TH, Ph: 020 8742 2605

ISSUE, 509 Aldridge Road, Great Barr, Birmingham B44 8NA, Ph: 0121 344 4414 (infertility support group)

Iyengar Yoga Institute, 223a Randolph Avenue, London WC2N 4HS, Ph: 020 7836 5220

La Leche League, Spencer Lester, 30 Whimbrel Way, Banbury, Oxon NW1 7YN, www.lalecheleague.org

Maternity Alliance, 59–61 Camden High Street, London NW1 7JL

Midwives Information and Resource Centre, 9 Elmdale Road,Clifton, Bristol BS8 1SL
Customer Services Ph: 0800 581009e-mail:- midirs@dial.pipex.com

Natracare Feminine Hygiene, c/- Bodywise (UK) Ltd, Bristol BS32 4DX Ph: 0145 461 5500, email: info@natracare.com (unbleached and chemical free tampons and pads)

Natural Parent, 4 Wallace Road, London N1 2PG, Ph: 0171 354 4592, email: wddty@zoo.co.uk (magazine for holistic family living)

Neils Yard Remedies, 15 Neals Yard, Covent Garden, London WC2H 9DP, Ph: 020 7379 7222, email: mail@nealsyardremedies.com (dried herbs and tinctures by mail order)

Nelsons Pharmacy, 73 Duke Street, London W1M 6BY, Ph: 020 7629 3118 (Bach flower remedies)

Organic Advisory Service, Elm Farm Research Centre, Hamstead Marshall, Berkshire RG20 0HR, Ph: 0148 365 7658, email: efrc@compuserve.com

Organic Growers Association, Aeron Park, Llangietho, Dyfed

Organic Information, PO Box 1503, Poole, Dorset BH14 8YE, Ph: 01202 715130

Portland Hospital for Women and Children, 205–209 Great Portland Street, London W1N 6AH, Ph: 0171 580 4400, Fax: 0171 631 1170

Society of Homoeopaths, 2 Artizan Road, Northampton NN1 4HU, Ph: 0160 462 1400

Society for the Promotion of Nutritional Therapy, PO Box 47, Heathfield, East Sussex TN21 8ZX, Ph: 0182 587 2921

Support after Termination for Abnormalities (SAFTA), 29 Soho Square, London W1V 6JB

The Ayurvedic Company of Great Britain, 50 Penywern Road, London SW5 9SX, Ph: 020 7370 2255

The BioElectric Shield, Natures Energy, Nine Elms, Swindon SN5 9UG, Ph: 0179 387 8637 (anti-radiation devices)

The British Acupuncture Council, Park House, 206–208 Latimer Road, London W10 6RE, Ph: 020 8964 0222

The British Chiropractic Association, 29 Whitley Street, Reading, Berkshire RG2 OE9, Ph: 0173 475 7557

The British Herbal Medicine Association, Sun House, Church Street, Stroud, Gloucestershire GL5 1JL, Ph: 0145 375 1389

The British Society for Mercury Free Dentistry, 1 Wellbeck House, 62 Wellbeck Street, London W1M 7HB, Ph: 020 7486 3127

The Dr Bach Foundation, Mount Vernon, Sotwell, Wallingford, Oxon OX10 OP2, Ph: 0149 183 4678 (Bach flower remedies)

The European Shiatsu Network, Highbanks, Lockeridge, Marlborough, Wiltshire SN8 4EQ, Ph: 0167 286 1362

The Green People Company, Brighton Road, Hardcross, West Sussex RH17 6BZ, Ph: 0144 440 1444 (mail order tinctures and environmentally safe, personal care products)

The Kinesiology Federation, PO Box 83, Sheffield S7 2YN, Ph: 0114 281 4064

The Moon Calendar Company, PO Box 2477, Bradford-on-Avon BA15 2XY, Ph: 0122 586 8850, www.mooncalendar.co.uk (lunar calendar)

The Natural Maid Company, Unit D7, Maws Craft Centre, Jackfield, Ironbridge, Shropshire TF8 7LS, Ph: 0195 288 3288, email: paint@livos.demon.co.uk (non-toxic paints and other products)

The Soil Association, Bristol House, 40–56 Victoria Street, Bristol BS1 6BY, Ph: 0117 929 0661, email: info@soilassociation.org

The Tai Chi Union for Great Britain, 69 Kilpatrick Gardens, Clarkston, Glasgow G76 7RF

Taoist Tai Chi Centre, Bounstead Road, Blackheath, Colchester, Essex C02 0DE, Ph: 1206 576167

Toxoplasmosis Trust, 61–71 Collier Street, London N1 9BE, Ph: 0171 713 0663

Vaginal Birth After Caesarean (VBAC) Support Group, 8 Wren Way, Farnborough, GU14 8SZ, Ph: 01252 543250

Vitamin Service, Dellrose Cottage, Littlewick Road, Knaphill, Woking, Surrey GU21 2JU, Ph: 01483 488845, Fax: 01483 799574

Wellbeing, The Health Research Charity for Women and Babies, 27 Sussex Place, Regents Park, London NW1 4SP, Ph: 020 7262 5337

Wholefood, 24 Paddington Street, London W1M 4DR

Recommended reading

Throughout this book we have referred to numerous studies and research. Although there is not room here to cite specific references, you will find all the relevant information in the books and journals recommended below. Specific inquiries can be directed to the authors c/- Transworld publishers.

Birth

Arms, S. *Immaculate Deception*, Bantam Books, USA, 1977.

Balaskas, J. *Active Birth*, Unwin Paperbacks, UK, 1983.

Balaskas, J. & Gordon, Y. *The Encyclopedia of Pregnancy and Birth*, Little, Brown & Company Limited, London, 1992.

Baldwin, R. *Special Delivery*, Les Femmes Publishing, Millbrae, 1979.

Edwards, M. & Waldorf, M. *Reclaiming Birth*, The Crossing Press, NY, 1984.

Fallows, C. *Having a Baby: The Essential Australian Guide to Pregnancy and Birth*, Doubleday, NSW, 1997.

Gaskin, I.M. *Spiritual Midwifery*, 3rd ed., The Book Publishing Company, Summertown, 1990.

Johnson, I. & P. *The Paper Midwife*, A.H & A.W. Reed Pty Ltd, Australia, 1980.

Katz Rothman, B. *In Labour—Women & Power in the Birthplace*, Junction Books, London, 1982.

Kitzinger, S. *The Experience of Childbirth*, Pelican Books, 1967.

Kitzinger, S. *Birth Over Thirty*, Penguin Books, USA, 1985.

Lidell, L. *The Book of Yoga*, Ebury Press, London, 1983.

Macfarlane, A. *The Psychology of Childbirth*, William Collins, Glasgow, 1977.

McCutcheon-Rosegg. *Natural Childbirth the Bradley Way*, E.P. Dutton Inc., NY, 1984.

Petty, R. *Home Birth*, Domus Books, Illinois USA, 1979.

Stoppard, Dr M. *New Pregnancy & Birth Book*, Viking, Ringwood, 1996.

Thomas, P. *Every Woman's Birthrights*, Thorsons, UK, 1996.

Birth (for children)

VanDam Anderson, S. & Simkin, P. *Birth—Through Children's Eyes*, Pennypress Inc., Washington USA, 1981.

Malecki, M. *Mom and Dad and I are Having a Baby*, Pennypress Inc., Washington USA, 1979.

Malecki, M. *Our Brand New Baby*, Pennypress Inc., Washington USA, 1980.

Bonding

Chilton Pearce, J. *Magical Child*, Bantam Books, USA, 1977.

Corkville Briggs, D. *Your Child's Self Esteem*, Dolphin Books, USA, 1975.

Janov, A. *The Feeling Child*, Sphere Books, UK, 1977.

Liedloff, J. *The Continuum Concept*, Penguin Books, Australia, 1986.

Montagu, A. *Touching*, Harper & Row, USA, 1971.

Sears, W. *Nighttime Parenting*, Dove Communications, Victoria, 1985.

Thevenin, Tine. *The Family Bed*, Avery Publishing Group Inc., NJ, USA, 1987.

Lifestyle/Environmental Factors

Foreman, R., Gilmour-White, S. & Forman, N. *Drug Induced Infertility and Sexual Dysfunction*, Cambridge University Press.

Powerwatch. *Living with Electricity*, Powerwatch, 2 Tower Road, Sutton, Ely, CB62QA Cambridgeshire, UK.

Foresight publications (available from Foresight Association—see Contacts & Resources)

The Adverse Effects of Alcohol on Reproduction

The Adverse Effects of Tobacco Smoking on Reproduction
The Adverse Effects of Lead
The Adverse Effects of Agrochemicals on Reproduction and Health
The Adverse Effects of Genito-urinary Infections

Nutrition

Sears, Barry. *Enter The Zone*, Harper Collins, NY, 1995.
Foresight publications (available from Foresight Association—see Contacts & Resources)
The Adverse Effects of Food Additives on Health
The Adverse Effects of Manganese Deficiency on Reproduction and Health
The Adverse Effects of Zinc Deficiency

Natural Remedies

Brightlight, Dr E.T. *Natural Childcare*, Brolga Publishing Pty Ltd, Ringwood, 1999.
Curtis, S. & Fraser, R. *Natural Healing For Women*, Pandora Press, London, 1991.
Howard, J. *Bach Flower Remedies for Women*, The C.W. Daniel Company Limited, Essex, 1992.
McQuade-Crawford, A. *Herbal Remedies for Women*, Prima Publishing, USA, 1997.
Northrup, Dr C. *Women's Bodies Women's Wisdom*, Judy Piatkus (Publishers) Ltd, London, 1998.
Ohashi, W. *Do-it-yourself Shiatsu*, Unwin Paperbacks, London, 1979.
Parvati, J. *Hygieia: A Woman's Herbal*, Freestone Collective, Berkeley, 1978.
Romm, A.J. *Natural Healing for Babies & Children*, The Crossing Press, Freedom, California, 1996.
Speight, P. *Homoeopathic Remedies for Women's Ailments*, Health Science Press, UK, 1985.
Tisserand, M. *Aromatherapy for Women*, 3rd ed., Thorsons, London, 1993.

Pregnancy

Cooper, D. *Your Baby, Your Way*, Random House Australia Pty Ltd, Milsons Point, 1999.

Eisenberg, A. Murkoff, H. & Hathaway, S. *What to Expect When You're Expecting*, Angus & Robertson, Sydney, 1987.

Griffey H. *The Really Useful A-Z of Pregnancy & Birth*, Thorsons, UK, 1996.

Kitzinger, S. *Being Born*, Collins, Sydney, 1986.

Kitzinger, S. & Bailey, V. *Pregnancy Day-By-Day*, Dorling Kindersley Limited, London, 1990.

Reid, E. & Elzer, S. *Maternity Reflexology—a guide for reflexologists*, Born to be Free & Soul to Sole Reflexology, Sydney, 1997.

Rodwell, L. & Kon, A. *Natural Pregnancy*, Salamander Books, London, 1997.

Romm, A.J. *The Natural Pregnancy Book*, The Crossing Press, Freedom, 1997.

Weed, S. *Wise Woman Herbal Childbearing Year*, Ash Tree Publishing, NY, 1986.

Wesson, N. *Morning Sickness*, Vermilion-Random House, London, 1997.

Recipe books

Alexander, S. *The Cook's Companion*, Penguin, Australia, 1997.

Airdre, G. *The Good Little Cookbook*, MacPlatypus Productions, Australia, 1998.

Hay & Bacon. *At My Table—Fresh & Simple*, Barbara Beckett, Australia, 1995.

Katzen, M. *Moosewood Cookbook*, Simon & Schuster, Australia, 1997.

Katzen, M. *Moosewood Restaurant Cooks at Home*, Simon & Schuster, Australia, 1994.

Katzen, M. *Moosewood Restaurant Kitchen Garden*, Simon & Schuster, Australia, 1992.

Katzen, M. *New Recipes from Moosewood Restaurant*, Simon & Schuster, Australia, 1997.

Katzen, M. *Sundays at Moosewood Restaurant*, Simon & Schuster, Australia, 1991.

Kilham, Chris. *The Whole Food Bible*, Inner Traditions, UK, 1997.

Milan, Lindley. *Plates*, New Holland, Australia, 1995.

Ombauer, Irma S. *The Joy of Cooking*, Simon & Schuster, Australia, 1998.

Solomon, Charmaine. *The Complete Asian Cookbook*, Lansdowne Publishing, Australia, 1992.

Solomon, Charmaine. *The Complete Vegetarian Cookbook*, Harper Collins, Australia, 1990.

Squirrels Cookbook, Squirrels Publishing, Brisbane, 1994.

Health issues from a holistic perspective

The following is a list of journals and newsletters which report on studies and research findings regarding health issues from a holistic perspective. Many of the studies we have mentioned have been reported in these journals.

Proof!; *What Doctors Don't Tell You*; and *Natural Parent* are all available from WDDTY, 77 Grosvenor Avenue, London, N5 2NN, Ph: 0171 354 4592, Fax: 0171 354 8907, email: wddty@zoo.co.uk

International Journal of Alternative & Complementary Medicine, Green Library, 9 Rickett Street, Fulham, London, Ph: 0171 385 0012, Fax: 0171 385 4566

Environment & Health News, The Environment Health Trust, PO Box 1954, Glastonbury, Somerset BA6 9FE, Ph: 0176 762 7038

Australian Journal of Medical Herbalism, Anne Cowper, PO Box 403, Morisset NSW 2264, Ph (02) 4973 4107, Fax: (02) 4973 4857

Health & Wellness Report, Tapestry Communications, Spectrum Marketing Services, PO Box 264, Toorak VIC 3142, Ph: (03) 8247 7938

Life Spirit, Tracey Harris, PO Box 312, Fortitude Valley QLD 4006, Ph: (07) 3854 1286

Herbalgram, American Botanical Council & Herb Research Foundation, PO Box 201660, Austin, Texas 78720 USA, Ph: (512) 331 8868

Alternative Medicine Digest, Future Medicine Publishing Inc. Editorial Office, 21 1/2 Main Street, Tiburon, California 94920 USA, Ph: (415) 789 8700

Australian Health & Healing, Australian Health Newsletters, PO Box 427, Paddington NSW 2021

Journal of Health Sciences, PO Box 6200, South Penrith NSW 2750

Alternative & Complementary Therapies, Mary Ann Leibert Inc,

2 Madison Avenue, Larchmart, NY 10538 USA, Ph: (914) 834 3100, Fax: (914) 834 3582

Journal of Nutritional & Environmental Medicine, Carfax Publishing Ltd, PO Box 25, Abingdon, Oxfordshire OX143UE UK

The Journal of the Australasian College of Nutritional & Environmental Medicine, ACNEM, 13 Hilton Street, Beaumaris VIC 3193, Ph: (03) 9589 6088, Fax: (03) 9589 5158

International Clinical Nutrition Review, Integrated Therapies, PO Box 370, Manly NSW 2095

Australasian Society of Oral Medicine and Toxicology, ASOMAT, PO Box A860, Sydney South NSW 2000, Ph: (02) 9867 1111, Fax: (02) 9665 5043

Soma Newsletter, PO Box 7180, Bondi Beach NSW 2026, Ph:(02) 9789 4805, Fax: (02) 9922 5747

Birthings, Homebirth Access Sydney, PO Box 66, Broadway NSW 2007

Birth Issues, CAPERS, PO Box 412, Red Hill QLD 4059, Ph: (07) 3369 9200, Fax: (07) 3369 9299

Index

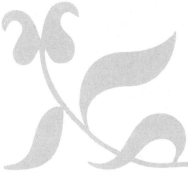